THE LOVEJOY KITCHEN

Transitioning to whole food, plant based eating
...and loving it!

ELISE LOVEJOY

Certified in Plant Based Nutrition

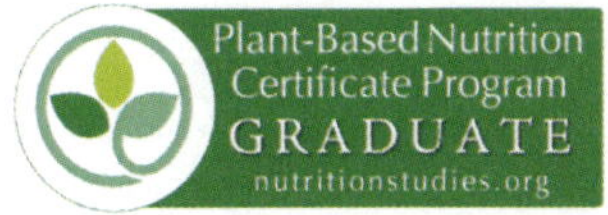

How to go whole food, plant based and still
enjoy many of your favorite foods.

By Elise Lovejoy

Published by The Lovejoy Kitchen Publishing.
For permissions, orders and other queries, contact the publisher at
thelovejoykitchen@gmail.com.

Book design by Kari Paine.

Featured photography by Dana Hursey Photography.

THE LOVEJOY KITCHEN, THE LOVEJOY KITCHEN PUBLISHING
and logo are trademarks of the author.

ISBN 978-1-7347153-0-9

AUTHOR'S NOTE

The Lovejoy Kitchen introduces you to preparing and eating whole and plant-based foods and provides recipes and other resources for those who wish to adopt a whole food, plant-based lifestyle.

This book does not provide medical or nutritional advice and does not take the place of a consultation with your own physician, nutritionist and other professional advisors. Not every food choice, recipe or supplement mentioned in this book is right for every reader. Your own health history, issues and conditions, allergies, medications and other factors must be considered when making food choices. For these reasons, you are strongly encouraged to consult your own professional health-care providers before using the information that I have shared here.

Although I feel that I have benefited from improvements in my health and well-being by changing what and how I eat, no guarantees can be made that you will have the same experience or that changing your diet will prevent or cure any condition or disease.

Elsewhere in this book, I have gratefully acknowledged and cited the physicians, researchers and others whose professional work I have studied. I have also acknowledged my certification by The Center for Nutrition Studies in its Plant-Based Nutrition Certificate Program. However, I want to make it clear to my readers that The Lovejoy Kitchen is solely my own work of authorship, and the book is not sponsored or endorsed by, and is not affiliated in any way with, those whom I have acknowledged and cited.

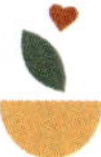

This cookbook is dedicated to all of the families who have lost a loved one too soon to a preventable illness, and to those who have found the courage to make these changes now.

I wish you strength, joy, and vibrant health as you begin this transition to the whole food, plant based food plan and lifestyle.

ACKNOWLEDGEMENTS

I am forever grateful to Dr. Dan Marcus in Santa Cruz, without whose whole food, plant based diet and lifestyle class I would not be on this food plan nor have written this cookbook.

To my dear friend Karen Moreno, who has been on this whole food, plant based (WFPB) journey with me since the beginning. Together, we have spent so many happy hours in the kitchen cooking and then sharing our WFPB meals.

To Richard Lovejoy for always believing in me and nudging me along when I faltered on this sometimes-daunting journey. He jumped into the whole food, plant based food plan with me and didn't look back, graciously eating all the different versions of my food and giving me honest feedback. A true friend, companion, and partner.

To Lexee Davis, my little sous chef. I do not know how I would have ever gotten all of these recipes tested without her help: she spent myriad hours chopping, slicing, and doing dishes—all with the best attitude and made the long days of recipe testing so much fun. She is the Lovejoy Kitchen's MVP!

To my super-talented and generous friend, Linda Kesler, who has always supported and encouraged me over the years. Her feedback on various aspects of the book, including the recipes, was immensely helpful.

To Kari Paine, who came up with the wonderful designs for the book and brought it all to life. I am very grateful that she took on this project.

To Dana Hursey whose beautiful photos are featured on the cover and at the beginning of each section in this book (except for Soups, Curries & Beans). I am grateful for his excellent work.

To Liza Baker whose coaching, feedback, and encouragement were an enormous help in completing this project. She is a health coach and the author of Flip Your Kitchen! a cookbook that teaches you how to plan and cook all of your meals from scratch, even with a busy schedule—an ideal skillset for transitioning to whole food, plant based eating.

To my wonderful daughter, Kelly Marie, for encouraging me and giving me her feedback on recipes and designs.

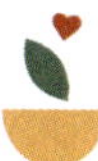

CONTENTS

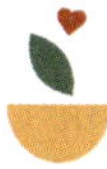

MY STORY

Like many of you, I have been searching for years for a food plan that optimizes my health, and also allows me to enjoy my favorite foods. For decades I had high cholesterol and was in and out of Type II diabetes. I spent years trying to figure out ways to lower my blood sugar and cholesterol. I was told to eat as little sugar as possible and increase my meat and fat intake. To my dismay, even when I adhered strictly to these recommendations, it didn't help much. And as I got older, my weight, blood sugar, and cholesterol gradually crept up. No matter what I did, I could not shift things in the right direction. I remember saying to a friend that, if I just knew what to eat to make myself healthy again, I would do it.

Then my husband and partner of 32 years was diagnosed with stage IV prostate cancer and I became even more motivated to find a food plan that really improved our health. I was lucky enough to take a class offered by my medical providers called Health and Wellness with a Whole-Food, Plant-Based Lifestyle. The doctors who taught the class had all been on this food plan for years. They showed us a plethora of research and data in support of the health benefits of the whole food, plant based (WFPB) diet. They also taught us which foods we could eat on the plan and gave us recipes and advice on setting up our own WFPB kitchen.

All of us had our blood pressure taken weekly by nurses at the class. By the end of the six weeks, all of the participants who stuck to the food plan saw their blood pressure go down significantly and those with Type II diabetes also noticed improvements in their blood sugar.

I have been eating WFPB for years now and continue to reap the benefits: my cholesterol is normal for the first time in decades, and my blood sugar is no longer in the diabetic zone. I am thirty pounds lighter, and at my ideal weight. I can run 3 miles a few times a week and I can do pushups and sit-ups. These are all things I never thought I would be able to do again. I don't crave sugar or have daily highs and lows, and I eat three meals and three snacks a day. I enjoy my food and enjoy cooking it and sharing it with family and friends. I would not go back to my old way of life and my old body for anything.

I feel so blessed to have finally found the answer, and I want to share it with you and show you how to make the transition and change your life. This is the cookbook I wish I'd had when I was transitioning to WFPB!

If you stick to eating a wholesome balance of the foods in this book, you will be making the transition, and you will experience the benefits.

After all, the most important thing in your life is your health!

WHOLE FOOD, PLANT BASED IN A NUTSHELL

Whole food, plant based eating includes consuming unrefined plant foods such as fruits, vegetables, whole grains, legumes, mushrooms, nuts, and seeds. It does not include meat, dairy products, or eggs, and eliminates or at least minimizes refined sugars, oils, and flours, added salt, and processed foods. A vegan diet is not necessarily whole food, plant based, because a vegan diet can include any foods as long as they have no meat, dairy, or other animal products in them.

WHY WHOLE FOOD, PLANT BASED?

Health

If adhered to properly, the WFPB food plan can lower blood pressure and blood sugar, promote weight loss, and reduce the risk of heart attack, stroke, and cancer. It can also reduce inflammation and improve autoimmune conditions. See the Resources (p 158) for more information on the research on the health benefits of WFPB eating.

Protecting the Environment

Not eating meat or dairy products decreases the need for commercial animal agriculture, which is a contributor to global warming as well as the destruction of waterways, rainforests and other wild lands.

Animal welfare

Not eating meat or dairy products decreases the demand for animals that have been raised in commercial feeding operations, which many people feel are inhumane.

The Research

I have studied in depth the research of Doctors T. Colin Campbell, Caldwell Esselstyn, John McDougall, Michael Gregor, Dean Ornish, Joel Fuhrman, and others who have all devoted much of their professional medical careers to studying and documenting the effects of the WFPB diet on cancer, heart disease, diabetes, and obesity among other medical conditions. See the Resources (p 158) for videos and books that explain their research in detail as well as other resources for individuals choosing the WFPB food plan and lifestyle. Each of these doctors has a different area of specialty, which gives them their own unique perspective, and they have drawn their own conclusions, which at times conflict with those of the others. Some of the doctors say no salt, and some say moderate amounts are okay; the same goes for nuts and avocados and even maple syrup and molasses. I have tried to strike a balance between the various opinions in developing the recipes for this cookbook. Most of these doctors have their own cookbooks or online recipes, which will be helpful if and when you are ready to transition to an even stricter WFPB food plan.

FOR PEOPLE WITH SERIOUS HEALTH CONDITIONS

This book is not intended to provide medical advice or replace the guidance of a medical professional. That being said, food is powerful medicine. If you have a serious or chronic health condition, talk to your doctor about your diet transition in case they want to monitor you and adjust your medications as necessary.

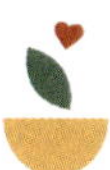

HOW TO USE THIS BOOK

This book is intended to help individuals who have decided to transition to a WFPB food plan. Eating 100% WFPB without allowing time to adjust can be so limiting that some people find they are unable to stick with the plan in the long term. Some doctors agree that eating WFPB 95% of the time is enough to provide major health benefits and is well worth doing. This means, for example, on occasion having a small amount of olive or avocado oil or eating something with a little refined flour or sugar. Allowing small amounts of these ingredients in your diet, at least temporarily, broadens the number of foods and meals you can eat and makes the transition easier.

Most of the recipes in this book are 100% whole food, plant based. However, some list ingredients that are okay in very small amounts, but not optimal, such as salt, avocado oil, and maple syrup. These are highlighted in italics in the recipes and often have a strict WFPB option noted. The goal is to eventually eliminate these foods entirely if you want to be on a strict WFPB food plan. The good news is that once you give up meat, dairy, and processed foods, your palate will change, and foods that you may not have liked at first will taste very good to you—even without added salt and sugar.

To paraphrase Dr. Joel Fuhrman from his book, *Eat to Live*, the goal is to eat the most nutrient dense foods as often as possible. For example, dark, leafy greens, cruciferous vegetables, and legumes are more nutrient dense than pasta, breads, or corn tortillas. When eating foods from this cookbook, it's important to include these nutrient-dense foods when eating starchy dishes with a lot of pasta or potatoes. Remember, when in doubt, always include beans and greens.

The most enjoyable way to eat WFPB is to mix and match flavors. For example, chili can be eaten on a bed of cornbread, topped with taco slaw, or salsa, guacamole, and black olives. Eat baked potatoes with chili, sour cream, and sliced green onions. Add the special sauce, lettuce, sliced tomatoes and onions to the veggie burgers, and throw green onion and jalapeño cornbread biscuits in the soups. Experiment with the sauces and suggested garnishes to make interesting flavor combinations. It's fun and delicious!

A great way to start your transition is to cook double batches of main courses or soups on the weekend and freeze the extra. After two or three weeks, you will have a good stash of frozen food for lunches and dinners. I cook big pots of oatmeal and freeze most of it, except for one container. Each morning, I heat some up in a small pot and add fruits, nuts, and seeds. See the Sample Meal Plan (p 156) for more ideas.

An added benefit of eating whole food, plant based is that you will discover you can eat a lot more than you imagined. These foods are usually lower in calories and much higher in nutrition than those of the standard American diet. A friend of mine started the food plan and was really sad that the scones from his favorite coffee shop were not on the food plan. So, he ate two scones with plant-based cream from this cookbook each day, in addition to other foods from this book. He lost 50 pounds in six months. He doesn't need to eat two scones a day anymore and is still on the food plan. I'm not advocating eating mostly desserts from this book, but if these treats help you with the transition and bring you joy, then by all means eat them. As your taste buds and body chemistry change, you will find yourself willingly letting go of foods you never thought you could live without. Relax, enjoy whatever you want to eat from this book and let the transition happen naturally.

Feel free to customize the recipes to your taste. As long as the ingredients you are using are WFPB, you should be making these foods to provide maximum enjoyment for yourself. Please note that ingredients in my recipes that also have a recipe in this cookbook are in title caps, followed by the page number of the recipe. You can also watch me make some of the recipes at The Lovejoy Kitchen on YouTube and on Instagram. And check out thelovejoykitchen. com for new recipes, cooking videos, resources, and a WFPB blog.

The bottom line is that, even if you only manage to eat 95% WFPB, you will notice significant benefits to your health. The key to transitioning is to take it in gradual, manageable chunks. For example, start by just changing to WFPB breakfasts and then switch over your snacks, then lunches, and finally include dinners. It is best to eat some salad and dark, leafy greens every day regardless of where you are in the transition. If you are able to stick to just eating the foods in this book, you will be making the transition. If the recipes in this book are as far as you can go, then enjoy...it will be good enough!

THE WHOLE FOOD, PLANT BASED LIFESTYLE

This way of eating is not just a food plan but a lifestyle. Choosing to eat WFPB means that, not only will you be making a lot of your own foods, but you will be very limited in the number and types of restaurants where you can eat. My recommendation is to find friends or family members who want to try it too, and to cook and eat together a few times a week. Cook double batches and freeze individual servings so you can take them to work with you or have them when you get home and don't feel like cooking. At first, it may feel overwhelming, but you will learn how to plan and cook meals that can last a few weeks if frozen and then augment with fresh salads and other quick and easy foods.

In order to get the most benefit from this lifestyle, it is important to include exercise and enough sleep in your daily routine. Most doctors recommend six to eight hours of sleep each night and at least moderate exercise, such as walking every day. Even if you just walk 15–20 minutes a day, that is a great start. You will find that, the longer you eat this way, the more energy you will have to work out and build your strength and fitness. Be patient with yourself and get at least moderate exercise and plenty of rest.

DINING OUT

Dining out on the WFPB food plan can be challenging. Many restaurants these days offer at least one vegan or vegetarian option, and salads or steamed vegetables and rice are also good choices. Vegetarian dishes often contain eggs or cheese and should be avoided or ordered without those ingredients. Many vegan meals contain refined flours and oils, so it's best to read the ingredients and make sure they are WFPB. If they contain a little oil or some refined flour, you can probably consume this on occasion without major consequences. You can also order a salad or a bowl (without meat, cheese or eggs) and get the dressing on the side. If you need a little dressing and it has some oil, this may be the best you can do for the time being. If I have to eat in a restaurant and cannot find anything that is whole food, plant based, then I go with the healthiest vegan option I can find. You can also bring small containers with WFPB salad dressing or non-dairy milk with you to restaurants. In general, it is best to keep dining out to a minimum, especially while you are transitioning to the WFPB food plan. The longer you have been on the food plan, the easier it is to navigate these situations.

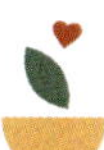

CHANGES TO EXPECT

My body has continued to change and adjust over the years since I started eating whole food, plant based. In the first few months, I lost weight and my blood pressure, blood sugar, and cholesterol dropped significantly. I also felt hungry a lot, which I addressed by eating WFPB meals and snacks as often as I needed. I noticed changes in my stools, including eliminating more often and more easily.

My body began to detox—releasing toxins stored from years of exposure to what we eat, drink, breath, and put on our skin. Symptoms of detoxing can last for weeks, depending on how bad your diet was before going WFPB. You can feel as though you have a mild flu—complete with queasiness, fatigue, and aches and pains—or just feel as though you are dragging a bit. People sometimes mistakenly think this is how they will feel long term on the WFPB food plan and quit. But don't give up! You will feel great. I have never felt better.

Finally, some people experience unexpected feelings and emotions as they move away from less healthy eating patterns and begin to take care of their body and see big changes. Whatever you experience, hang in there. If you stick to the food plan, you will experience changes to your body and your health that most of us long ago gave up on ever achieving.

REDUCING YOUR TIME IN THE KITCHEN

Eating whole food, plant based requires more time in the kitchen than eating at restaurants, fast food places, or buying processed meals and snacks. It is important to be strategic about how much time you spend in the kitchen. Cook as much as you can in large quantities and freeze or refrigerate it. Soups, chili, sauces, naan bread, biscuits, and scones can all be cooked in double batches and frozen. I make a large salad a couple of times a week and leave the dressing off so that it lasts me 3–4 days. I also make a big batch of taco slaw at least once a week to put on chili, quesadillas, nachos, and green salad. Once you get in the habit of cooking in quantity and freezing or refrigerating the food, you will find that you have a wonderful variety of your favorite WFPB dishes available to you whenever you want them. Everything worth having is worth working for and your health is the most precious gift you have.

EQUIPMENT

There is some equipment that will definitely make your life easier and food preparation quicker on this food plan. Helpful or necessary equipment in the recipes will be listed in the Equipment box. I use the following regularly when cooking these recipes:

- Airfryer
- Baking sheets
- Bread machine
- Bullet-style blender with small and large receptacles
- Electric nonstick griddle
- Food processor
- Glass storage containers with lids that seal

- Immersion blender
- Mortar and pestle
- Parchment paper
- Pizza stone
- Rolling pin
- Electric salad slicer
- Wooden pizza peel
- Spray bottle for water

INGREDIENTS

Be Choosy

Vegan foods can vary greatly in ingredients and quality. Many of them contain ingredients that should be avoided. As always, it is best to make your own, but many of us do not have the time for this, so, for the following products, I have suggested ingredients to look for and those to avoid.

Non-dairy milks (soy, almond, cashew, oat, coconut, pea)
- Look for: organic, non-GMO ingredients
- Avoid: carrageenan, flavorings, oils, sweeteners, added calcium, emulsifiers

Nutritional yeast (sometimes in refrigerator in health food stores)
- Look for: organic, non-GMO ingredients
- Avoid: fortified with vitamins/minerals

Hummus
- Look for: organic, non-GMO ingredients
- Avoid: oil as the second or third ingredient, guar gum, potassium sorbate, flavorings

Bread
- Look for: organic, non-GMO ingredients, sprouted grains, other grains and seeds in addition to wheat
- Avoid: sugar, sweeteners, oils, dough conditioners, preservatives

Soy products (stick to tofu and tempeh only)
- Look for: organic, non-GMO ingredients
- Avoid: processed meat substitutes (soy sausages, bacon, etc.), oil as one of the first ingredients, flavorings, MSG

Sauces (Worcestershire sauce, etc.)
- Look for: organic, non-GMO ingredients
- Avoid: oil as one of the first ingredients, guar gum, potassium sorbate, flavorings, MSG, fish

Veggie broth
- Look for: organic, non-GMO ingredients, filtered water, low sodium
- Avoid: oil, MSG, flavorings

Salsas
- Look for: organic, non-GMO ingredients
- Avoid: oil, sugar, MSG, whey protein concentrate

Oils
- Look for: organic, non-GMO, avocado oil for high heat, olive oil for lower or no heat
- Avoid: cottonseed, grapeseed, canola, soybean, and corn oil

Vinegars
- Look for: organic, non-GMO
- Avoid: potassium sorbate, flavorings

Spices
- Look for: organic, non-GMO
- Avoid: MSG, flavorings, anticaking agents

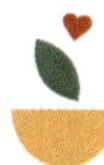

INGREDIENTS, CONTINUED

Fruits and Veggies

The WFPB food plan should include as many organic ingredients as possible. In fact, the recipes in this book do not specify that the ingredients are organic because it is recommended that *all ingredients be organic*. Organic foods are grown without the use of synthetic fertilizers or pesticides and are always non-GMO. If you cannot obtain organic ingredients, don't give up. The health benefits of this food plan will still be significant even with conventionally grown food.

Listed below are the fruits and vegetables that get treated with the most synthetic pesticides, herbicides, and fertilizers according to www.ewg.org and www.foodnews.org. It is advisable to get the following ingredients organic if at all possible.

- Strawberries
- Spinach
- Nectarines
- Apples
- Peaches
- Pears
- Cherries
- Grapes
- Celery
- Tomatoes
- Sweet bell peppers
- Potatoes

Sweeteners

On the strict WFPB food plan, all sugars except ground up whole dates or date sugar should be avoided. That includes maple syrup, agave syrup, and all variations of refined sugar and corn syrup. However, the transitional food plan allows for a very small amount of maple syrup or agave syrup. There are different opinions on which is better—I personally use maple syrup. Date sugar is simply ground up whole dates that are dried, which is technically acceptable on the stricter food plan. You can use this if you want to, but you will need to use a lot to achieve the same level of sweetness that a small amount of maple or agave syrup provides.

Salt

On an ideal food plan, we can get enough salt from the food we eat. Recommendations about salt intake vary greatly depending on the expert. Some believe that no salt should be added to any food. Doctors who are treating patients with heart disease—especially high blood pressure—recommend a very low salt intake, and all of the experts recommend keeping salt intake moderate. For the purposes of transitioning to eating WFPB, I include some salt in the recipes, with the recommendation to taper it off as your taste buds adjust. Again, if the prospect of having your food be so bland that it is unenjoyable is preventing you from committing to the food plan, then it is probably better to add some salt to your food. The best way to do this is to add salt at the table rather than during cooking, which will give you more flavor using less salt.

Refined Oils

Moving away from refined oils is an important part of the WFPB food plan. This includes not only avoiding deep fried foods, but also minimizing or avoiding using oil in cooking like sautéing or roasting as well as on salads. It is very difficult to avoid all refined oil, especially if one is traveling or eating out. It is probably better for you to eat a salad with a small amount of oil than no salad at all. If you must, use the smallest amount possible of olive oil along with vinegar. Many people are able to transition to just using balsamic vinegar on their salads. I squeeze lime juice onto my salad; some people use lemon juice. This book also has recipes for oil free fruit, miso and tahini dressings.

The best way to sauté vegetables is with water. Instead of using oil, sprinkle a little water in the pan as the vegetables are cooking on a medium heat. Don't use too much water, otherwise the vegetables will boil. Keep adding small amounts of water as needed. It is a bit of an adjustment, but once you get the hang of it, you will find that it works just fine, even for caramelizing onions. You can also use vegetable broth for sautéing instead of water. If you need to use a little oil in high heat cooking, avocado oil is best suited for this.

Non-dairy Milks

There is a lot of debate about which is the best non-dairy milk to drink. The most common options are soy, almond, oat, pea, coconut, and cashew. Soy milk has the most protein. It also has other important nutrients like isoflavones and it works well for cooking and baking. Pea milk has the next most protein. When selecting a non-dairy milk, make sure it is organic or at least non-GMO, unsweetened, and without oil, carrageenan, or other additives. All of the milks listed above are acceptable on the transitional WFPB food plan.

Herbs and Spices

Herbs and spices have high levels of nutrients and antioxidants. They can help detox your body as well as reduce the risk of heart disease, cancer, and diabetes. See the Resources (p 158) for where to find more info on this. Try to add herbs and/or spices to every meal. I put cinnamon on my oatmeal in the morning and have cilantro in my salads throughout the day. Add ginger and turmeric to stir fries and curries, and make Lovejoy Golden Milk for a warm and delicious dose of spices.

Soaked Cashews

A number of the recipes in this book call for soaked cashews I find it is easiest to buy a pound of raw organic cashews or cashew pieces, soak them for at least two hours, drain, and then freeze them in a resealable gallon freezer bag, so I have soaked cashews any time I need them. Keep in mind cashews, like all nuts, are high in calories. If your main focus is to lose weight, keep the nut-based creams to a minimum.

Boosting your Protein

While green vegetables, legumes, and tubers already provide a lot of protein, you can further boost your protein by adding hemp seed, freshly ground flax seed, and walnuts to your oatmeal, drinking soy milk instead of almond or oat milk, and including nuts and seeds in your snacks and on your salads. Add garbanzo beans and other legumes to salads and soups, and add tofu, tempeh, and mushrooms to stir fries and other dishes.

SNACKS

Transitioning to the WFPB food plan is a big change for your body. Since plant based whole foods are generally lower in calories than meat, dairy products, and processed foods, you may find yourself feeling hungry during the transition. Don't worry, once you are fully on the food plan, you will find yourself feeling more satisfied from your food than you ever have. You won't feel sluggish after you eat anymore or be on a roller coaster of sugar highs and lows.

It is important to "arm yourself with food," especially if you are going to work or will be out running errands for a while. If you always have WFPB snacks to eat, you will be far less tempted to grab something out of desperation that is off the food plan. In general, starchy whole foods are the most filling and can make great snacks. For example, white potatoes and sweet potatoes are complete foods and can be eaten in many forms to fill you up. They are very low calorie and have a lot of nutrients. Just make sure you are not eating them with oils or other fats. Here are a few snack suggestions (asterisks indicate recipes from this book):

- Fresh vegetables (carrots, bell peppers, cucumber, broccoli, cauliflower) with Hummus* or other dips.
- Baked Potato* with Sour Cream* and sliced green onions
- Mashed Potatoes* with peas and/or corn
- Air Fried French Fries* or Sweet Potato Fries*
- Baked, roasted, or mashed sweet potato
- Raw, organic brazil nuts (it is recommended that people who do not eat meat eat a small amount of these nuts each week as a reliable source of selenium)
- *Mary's Gone Crackers* brand or other WFPB crackers with Hummus*

- Pumpkin Nuggets*
- Dried apples (no sulfites)
- Avocado Toast* with WFPB bread
- Veggie Toast with Hummus* with WFPB bread
- Puffed wheat or other grains with non-dairy milk
- GoRaw sprouted pumpkin or sunflower seeds or tamari pumpkin seeds
- Scones* or Biscotti*
- Fresh fruit
- Oatmeal* with fresh fruit
- Homemade tortilla chips* with fresh salsa* or guacamole*

WHEN YOU'RE DESPERATE FOR TREATS

Sometimes for either physical or emotional reasons, we crave food that is not whole food, plant based. I have found that eating unsweetened dried mango, dates, or prunes, a small amount of dark chocolate (over 70% cocoa) with nuts, Scones*, Biscotti*, or other desserts from the book can help satisfy these cravings. If you eat something that is not WFPB, do not give up. Transitioning is a process. Pick yourself up, dust yourself off and recommit.

The more you eat on the WFPB food plan, the less you will crave meat, dairy, and processed and sugary foods. Many people eventually find that eating foods that are not WFPB makes them feel sick since they are no longer used to eating the sugars, oils, and saturated fats. You are making a choice to transform your health and your life. Be patient with yourself and keep focused on the benefits that will inevitably come with this transition.

COFFEE

Many people ask if coffee is included in the whole food, plant based food plan. There is a broad array of opinions on this. Most doctors whose focus is to treat patients with heart disease do not include any kind of caffeinated drinks in the food plan. Others feel that drinking coffee perpetuates the "pleasure trap" and should be avoided for this reason. Still others feel that it is a plant based drink and, if consumed in moderation with non-dairy milks and no sweeteners or very small amounts of maple or agave syrup will not cause harm. If the prospect of giving up coffee is stopping you from fully committing to the WFPB food plan and lifestyle, then it is definitely better for you to include moderate amounts of coffee and commit to the food plan. After being on the food plan for a while, you will almost certainly feel more energetic and begin to lose cravings for stimulants like sugar and coffee. That may be a good time to reconsider whether you need coffee in your daily routine and think seriously about replacing it with green tea or other beverages.

ALCOHOL

A strict WFPB food plan does not include alcohol. However, the process of transitioning away from less healthy foods and beverages can be undertaken gradually. When I started eating WFPB, I had about one drink a week. I didn't worry about it too much and found that, as my health improved, I did not want to drink as much. I felt great and after a while, replacing an alcoholic drink with a Pomegranate Mint Sparkler* or one of the other delicious beverages in this cookbook became preferable. I think it is much easier to let the process of reducing or eliminating alcohol consumption happen organically as your body feels better.

REQUIRED SUPPLEMENTS

According to most of the doctors listed in the Resources (p 158), the only supplement you should need on a WFPB food plan is vitamin B12. I take a 1000 mg capsule once a week. Most of the doctors on whose research this cookbook is based recommend against using any other supplements and instead suggest getting the nutrients you need from the foods you eat.

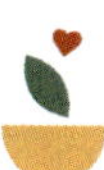

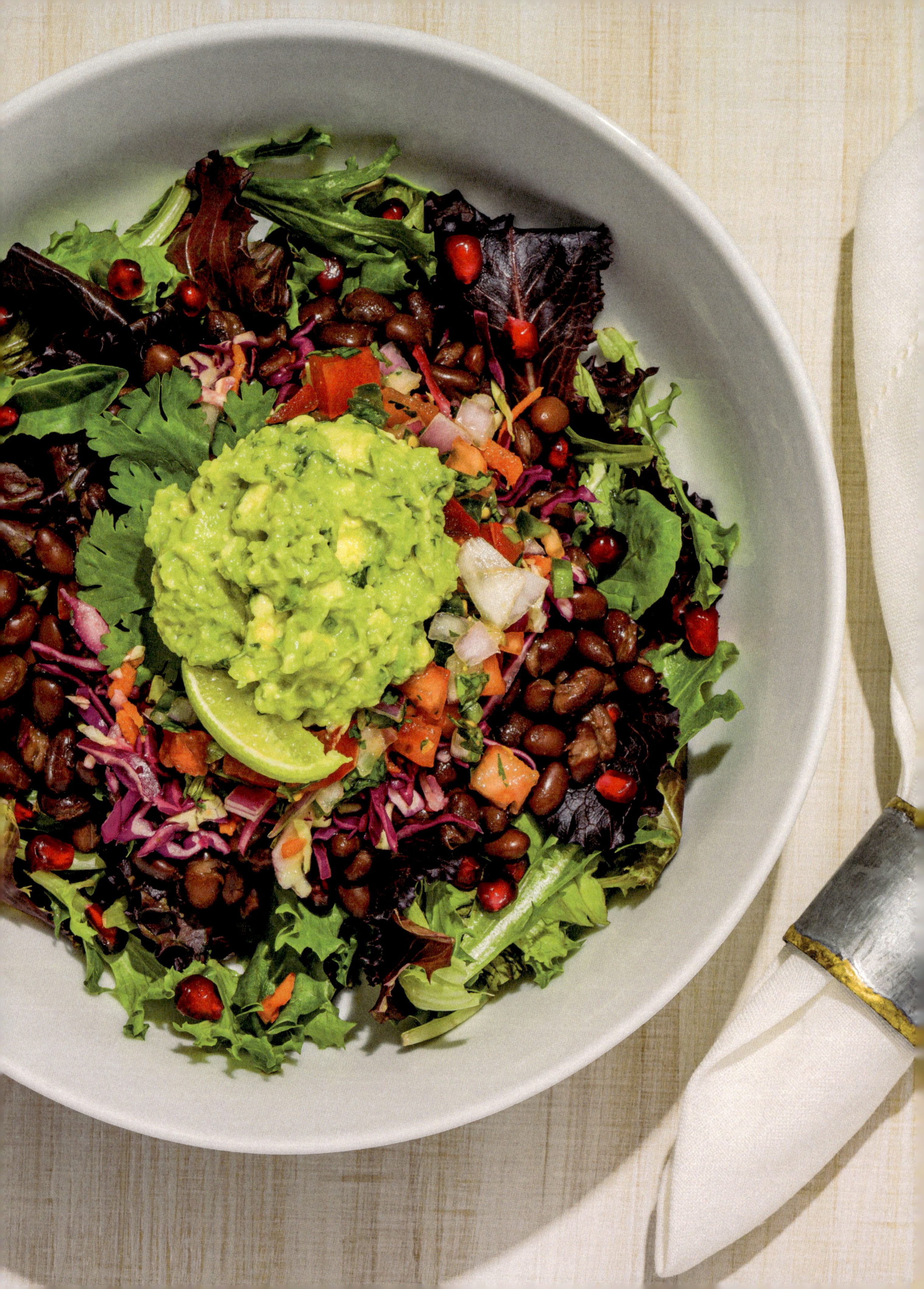

SALADS

Salads are a delicious staple of the whole food, plant based food plan. I have one to two salads per day. My favorite is always the farmers market salad with seasonal fruit, topped with a good helping of taco slaw and sprinkled with fresh lime juice. I also put the taco slaw on my southwestern soups, chili, nachos, and other dishes. Feel free to experiment with your favorite fruits and vegetables to make salads that suit your tastes. Remember, it's best to use as many organic ingredients as possible.

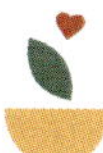

FALL KALE SALAD

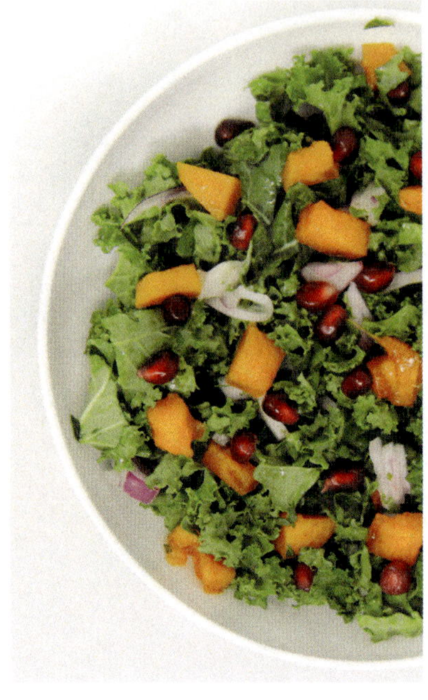

This colorful, nutrient-packed salad is great for parties and potlucks. The pomegranate seeds are tart and refreshing, and the persimmon adds a sweet flavor.

¼ cup fresh lemon juice

¼ tsp *maple syrup* (optional, eventually omit)

1 bunch curly leaf kale, stripped of the stems and finely chopped, (about 8 cups, loosely packed)

½ cup thinly sliced red onion

⅓ cup pomegranate seeds

¾ cup diced, ripe fuyu persimmon

2 tbsp raw or toasted pumpkin seeds

servings

6

1. Mix the lemon juice and maple syrup in a small bowl.

2. Toss the liquid with the finely chopped kale and red onions and let sit for an hour, stirring occasionally.

3. When ready to serve, add the persimmon, pomegranate and pumpkin seeds.

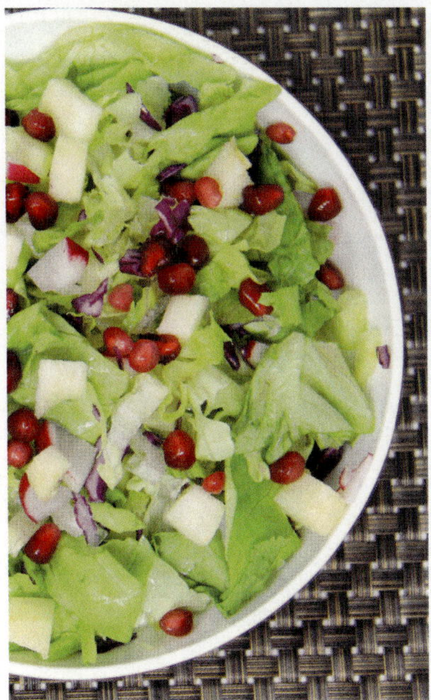

servings

6

FARMERS MARKET SALAD

This salad is fun to make right after going to the farmers market. The sweetness and tanginess of the fruit make this a delicious salad to eat even with very little dressing. I like to put Taco Slaw (p 28) on top of it for extra crunch and zest. If you don't have a farmers market nearby, many stores now carry living lettuces, which are sold still on the root ball. Regular lettuce is fine, too. Try adding other fruits and veggies like jicama, chopped snap peas, beets, mango, etc.

If you are making this salad to last a few days in the refrigerator, then do not add the tomato or avocado except to the serving you are about to eat. This way, they won't get soggy. I usually eat a salad this size over 2–3 days.

1 head red or green butter lettuce (baby lettuces can be used, too), washed and chopped

1 heart of romaine lettuce, washed and finely chopped

1–2 cups chopped baby spinach (optional)

1 cup thinly sliced red cabbage (optional)

1 grated carrot

¾ cup diced cucumber

3 radishes diced

1 ripe tomato, diced (optional, when in season)

½ avocado, diced (optional)

1 ripe pear or apple, diced (spring/summer) or 1 fuyu persimmon, diced (fall/winter)

⅓ cup fresh pomegranate seeds

1. Combine all ingredients in a large salad bowl.

2. Serve with any of the salad dressings listed in the Dips, Sauces, and Dressings section of this cookbook or your own WFPB creation.

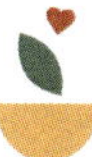

NACHO SALAD

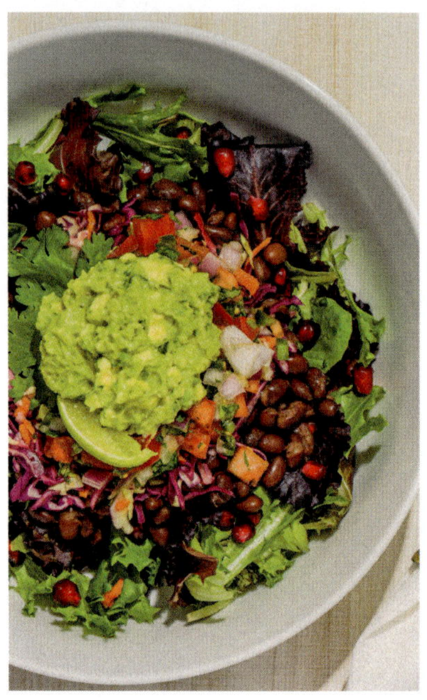

This is a delicious alternative to Nachos (p 58) on a hot day. If you already have the salads, Guacamole, and Salsa made, it only takes a few minutes to throw together. Try eating with Homemade Tortilla Chips (p 70).

3–4 cups Farmers Market (p 25) or other green salad

2 cups Taco Slaw (p 28)

1 can spicy black beans (1 ½ cups Spicy Black Beans [p 122]), rinsed and drained

1 cup Guacamole (p 95)

1 cup Salsa (p 101)

1 lime for juicing

Salt and pepper to taste (eventually omit salt)

4 sliced green onions for garnish

servings

2 large bowls

1. In two individual salad bowls, layer the taco slaw on top of the green salad.

2. Top with black beans (heated or room temperature), guacamole, and salsa.

3. Sprinkle with lime juice and add salt and pepper to taste.

4. Garnish with sliced green onions.

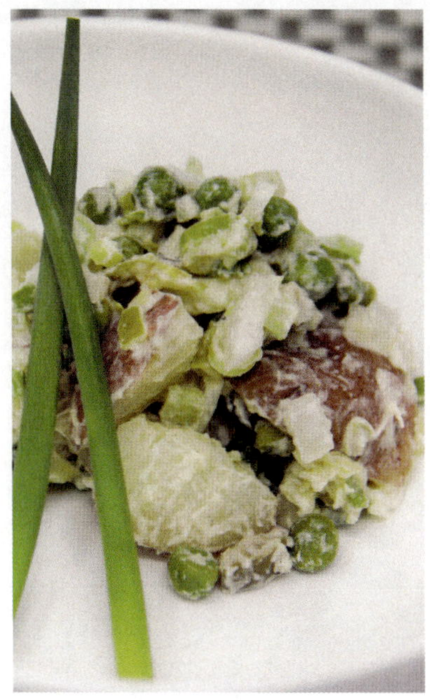

POTATO SALAD

Potatoes are a complete food, and the peas give this hearty salad an extra boost of protein. I like to make it with baby red potatoes with the skin on but russet or Yukon Gold are fine, too. Eat it as a main course along with Watermelon Mint Salad (p 29) or a green salad or as a side with Veggie Burgers (p 62). This salad is even better the next day.

If possible, try to buy organic pickles, olives and pepperoncinis and read the ingredients. They should ideally contain the vegetable, water, sea salt, herbs, distilled vinegar and citric acid. I try to avoid products with other preservatives.

servings

6–8

6 cups diced potatoes

¾ cup Sour Cream (p 102)

1 tbsp yellow mustard (or to taste)

Salt and pepper to taste (eventually omit salt)

3 celery stalks, finely chopped

1 cup frozen peas

½ cup finely chopped red or sweet onion

¼ cup finely diced pepperoncinis (optional if you like spicy)

¼ cup finely chopped black olives (optional)

¼ cup finely chopped dill pickles (optional, leave out to reduce salt)

¼ cup finely chopped green onions

1. Bring the diced potatoes to a boil in a large pot of water. Then simmer for 10–15 minutes or until the potatoes are just tender when pierced with a knife. Do not let them get mushy.

2. Meanwhile, in a medium bowl, mix the mustard with the sour cream and add salt (optional) and pepper.

3. When they are cooked, drain and cool the potatoes.

4. Mix the potatoes with the other vegetables and stir in the sour cream mixture.

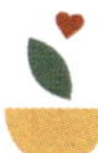

TACO SLAW

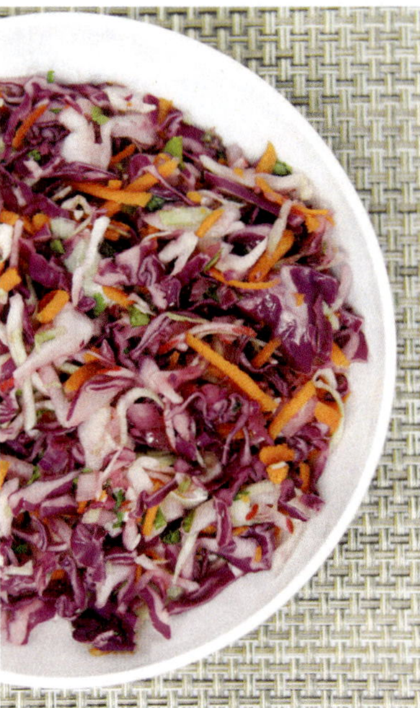

This tangy salad is a wonderful addition to any southwestern dish, such as Nachos (p 58), Bean and Cheese Quesadillas (p 53), or Black Bean and Corn Chili (p 40). It is also delicious mixed in with the Farmers Market Salad (p 25). I always have it have it in my refrigerator along with green salad. Using an electric salad slicer to slice the cabbage and grate the carrots and radishes saves a lot of time.

3 cups finely sliced red cabbage

3 cups finely sliced green cabbage

1 large carrot, grated (1 cup)

3 large radishes, grated (½ cup)

½ cup chopped cilantro

¼ cup red onion or sweet onion, finely minced (optional)

1 tbsp jalapeno finely minced (optional)

Juice of 2 limes (about ¼ cup or to taste)

Salt and pepper to taste (eventually omit salt)

Green onions for garnish

servings

4–6

equipment

Electric salad slicer (optional)

1. Mix all of the ingredients thoroughly in a bowl with lime juice and salt (optional) and pepper and let sit 15 minutes before serving.

2. Garnish with sliced green onions.

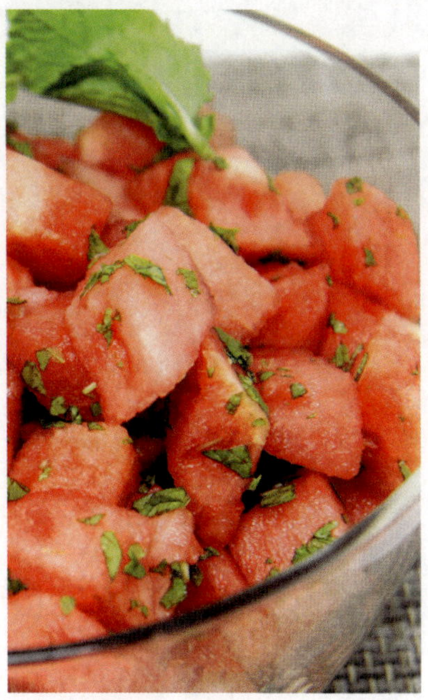

WATERMELON MINT SALAD

This refreshing dish is wonderful as a side with Potato Salad (p 27) and Veggie Burgers (p 62) or just on its own to cool down on a hot day.

6 cups cubed ripe watermelon

¼ cup finely minced fresh spearmint leaves

servings

6

1. In a large bowl, mix the spearmint in with the chopped watermelon.

2. Let sit a few minutes before serving.

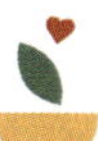

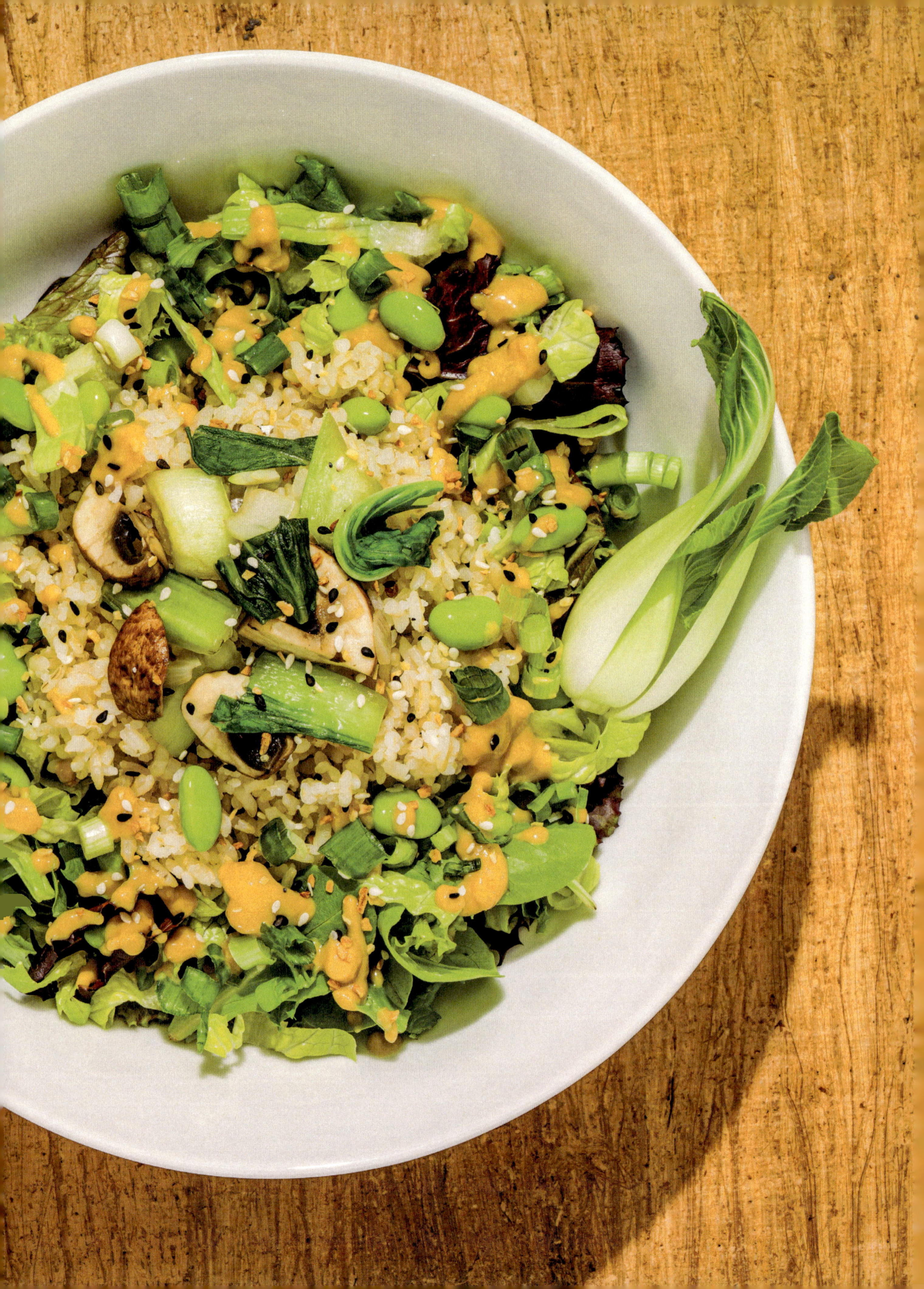

BOWLS

Bowls are a fantastic way to keep variety in your food plan and easily assemble custom WFPB meals. If you have an Instant Pot, you can quickly make a lot of the grains and legumes for them in large quantities and freeze them. If you don't have time to make these from scratch, then you can buy them at most grocery stores frozen, canned, or packaged. It is preferable to buy low-sodium products. Assemble your bowls using at least one item from each category below, and do not limit yourself to these items. Bowls are also a great way to use leftovers.

Greens	Grains	Legumes	Vegetables	
Arugula	Barley	Beans	Avocado	Corn
Baby Greens	Brown Rice	Lentils	Bok Choy	Eggplant
Baby Lettuces	Buckwheat	Peanuts	Broccoli	Mushrooms
Kale	Bulgur	Peas	Cabbage	Plantains
Lettuce	Millet	Tempeh	Cauliflower	Potatoes
Microgreens	Quinoa	Tofu	Carrots	Sweet Potatoes
Spinach	Wild Rice			
Sprouts				

Seeds/Nuts	Herbs/Spices		Dressings	
Chia	Basil	Mint	Balsamic vinegar	Salsa (p 101)
Ground flax	Cayenne	Parsley	Harissa	Sriracha
Hemp	Cilantro	Pepper flakes	Korean Hot Sauce (p 98)	Tahini Dressing (p 104)
Pumpkin	Coriander	Turmeric	Miso Dressing (p 99)	Tamari
Sunflower	Cumin		Peanut Sauce (p 97)	Tzatziki (p 105)
Sesame	Dulse flakes			
Watermelon	Ginger			

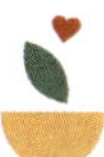

ASIAN BOWL

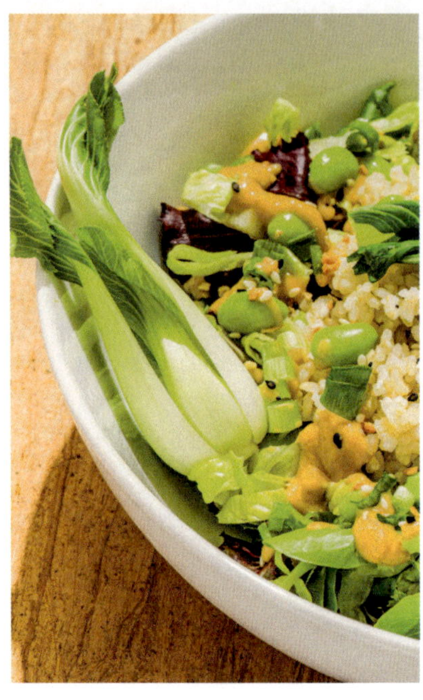

This zesty bowl is packed with protein and leafy greens. Feel free to add marinated tofu for additional protein.

¼ cup diced onions

1 small baby bok choy

½ cup sliced mushrooms

2 cups baby greens

½ cup finely sliced Napa cabbage

¾ cup brown or wild rice

2 tbsp cooked, peeled edamame (fresh or frozen soy beans)

1 tsp toasted sesame seeds

A sprinkle of dulse/seaweed flakes

1 tbsp sliced green onions

A light drizzle of Miso Dressing (p 99) and/or Korean Style Hot Sauce (p 98)

servings

1 large bowl

1. Water sauté the onions for 2 minutes, then add the baby bok choy and mushrooms and sauté for 2–3 minutes more.

2. In a large bowl, layer the baby greens, then the cabbage, the rice, and then the bok choy/mushroom mixture.

3. Top with the edamame, sesame seeds, seaweed flakes, and sliced green onions. Drizzle with Miso Dressing and/or Korean Style Hot Sauce.

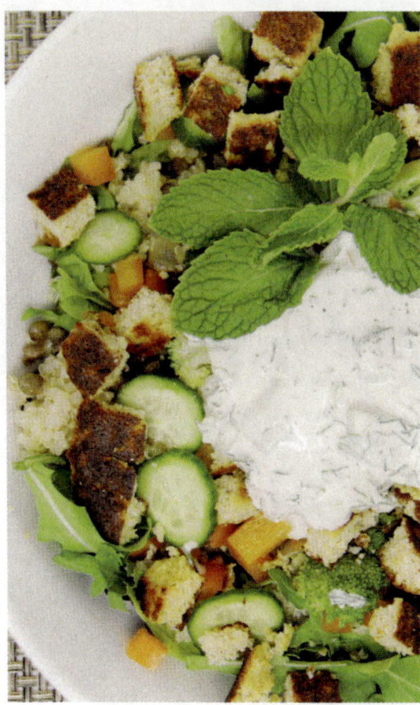

MIDDLE EASTERN BOWL

I love this hearty bowl. The falafel makes it extra filling. My favorite dressing for this is the Tzatziki.

servings

1 large bowl

¼ cup diced shallots or onions

1 cup small broccoli florets

2 cups chopped lettuce and arugula (or greens of your choice)

¾–1 cup cooked bulgur or quinoa

½ cup cooked lentils

Orange or yellow pepper slices to taste

Sliced cucumber to taste

1 Falafel (p 55) patty cut into small pieces

1 tbsp dried currants or finely chopped Turkish dried apricots

1 tbsp chopped parsley (omit if you use Tzatziki)

2 tsp chopped mint (omit if you use Tzatziki)

Tzatziki (p 105), Tahini Dressing (p 104), and/or harissa paste

1. Water sauté the shallots or onion and broccoli florets for 4–5 minutes or until the broccoli is tender when pricked with a knife. Set aside to cool.

2. Layer everything in the bowl, starting with the lettuce and going down the ingredients list, adding the sautéed vegetables with the pepper and cucumber slices.

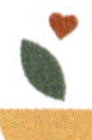

SOUTHWESTERN BOWL

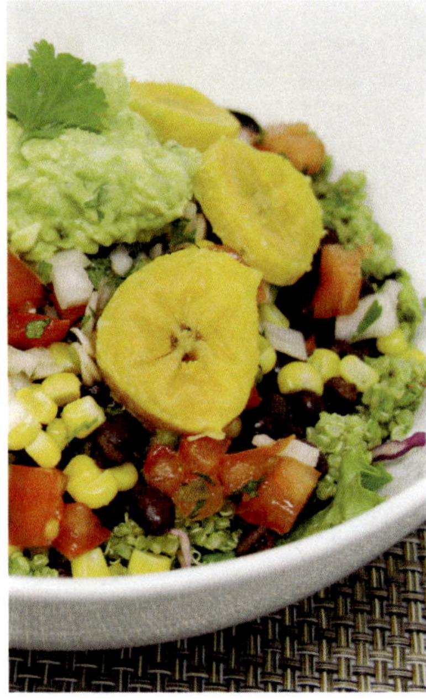

This filling and flavorful bowl is one of my favorites. The Green Quinoa adds a great flavor and texture and the sweet potatoes or plantains add sweetness to balance the zing of the Taco Slaw and Salsa. I like to put 6 slices of steamed plantain on each bowl.

1 small sweet potato or 1 ripe plantain

2 cups baby lettuces

¾ cup Taco Slaw (p 28)

¾–1 cup Green Quinoa (p 69)

½–¾ cup Black Beans, canned or homemade, (p 119) (spicy optional), rinsed and drained

¼ cup frozen corn, thawed, or canned corn, rinsed and drained

¼–⅓ cup sliced avocado or Guacamole (p 95)

¼ cup Salsa (p 101)

1 tbsp chopped, fresh cilantro (optional)

servings

1 large bowl

1. Peel and cut a small sweet potato into little chunks or chop a ripe plantain into 2-inch slices (with the peel on) and place them in a steamer basket in a medium pot with about an inch of water in the bottom. Steam for 10–15 minutes or until tender when pricked with a knife. Set aside to cool.

2. When cooled, peel the plantain pieces (if using) and cut into ¼-inch slices.

3. In a large bowl, layer the baby lettuce, Taco Slaw, Green Quinoa, Black Beans, sweet potatoes or plantains, and sweet corn. Then top with sliced avocado or Guacamole, Salsa, and fresh cilantro.

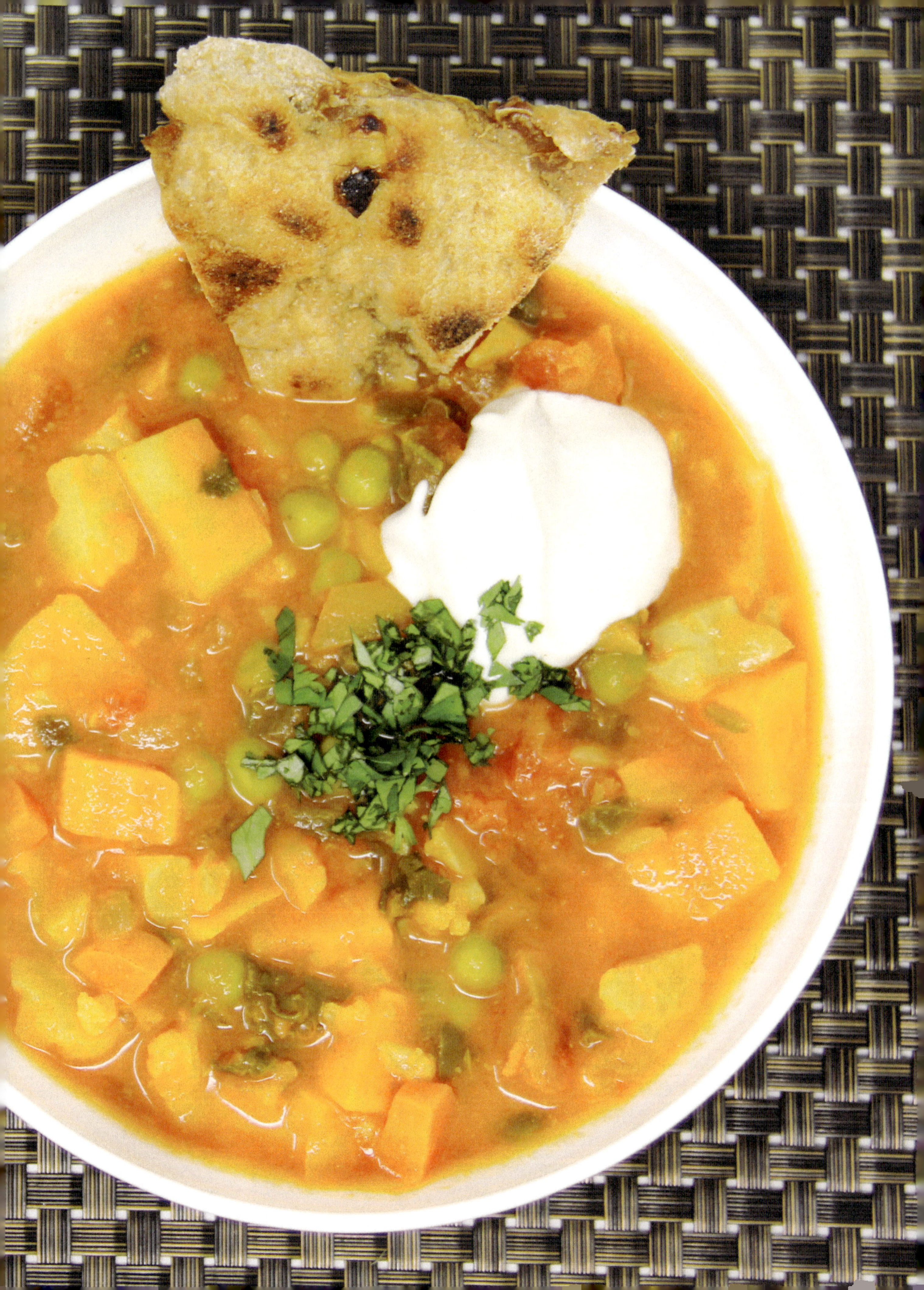

SOUPS, CURRIES & BEANS

Soups and curries are a fantastic way to get a wonderful variety of highly nutritious foods in one bowl. They are easy to make in large batches and freeze in small servings to take for lunches. They can be enjoyed with a green salad, green onion and jalapeño cornbread biscuits, caramelized onion naan bread, savory cornbread, and homemade tortilla chips to name a few. They are easy to customize by adding your own favorite vegetables, herbs, and spices.

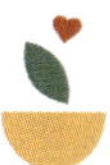

ASIAN STYLE MUSHROOM NOODLE SOUP

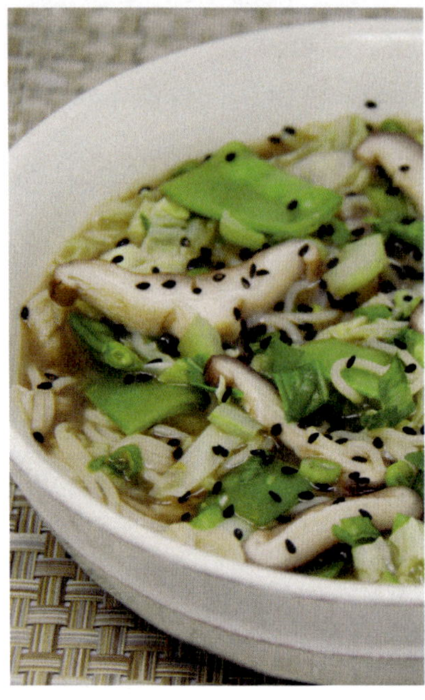

The crisp vegetables and tender noodles make this soup delicious. Because of this, I prefer to only make enough for one meal and avoid having leftovers. Garnish this soup with chopped fresh green onions and toasted black sesame seeds or seaweed flakes.

8 cups mushroom broth

2 large garlic cloves, pressed

2 tsp fresh grated ginger

2 tbsp tamari, preferably low salt

1 tsp tahini

¼ tsp red pepper flakes, optional

4 blocks of brown rice and quinoa ramen noodles (10–12 oz)

1 cup snow peas, ends cut off and cut in half

1 cup snap peas, strings removed and cut in half

2 cups thinly sliced green cabbage (Napa or savoy is best)

2 baby bok choy, sliced

2 cups sliced crimini or shitake mushrooms

Toasted black sesame seeds and/or seaweed flakes for garnish

Sliced green onions for garnish

servings

About 6

1. Pour mushroom broth into a large pot.

2. Add garlic, ginger, tamari, tahini, and chili flakes, if using, and bring to a boil.

3. Add ramen noodles and cook for 2 minutes, pulling the noodles apart with a fork after the first minute.

4. Add all of the vegetables and cook for 2 more minutes. Garnish and serve right away.

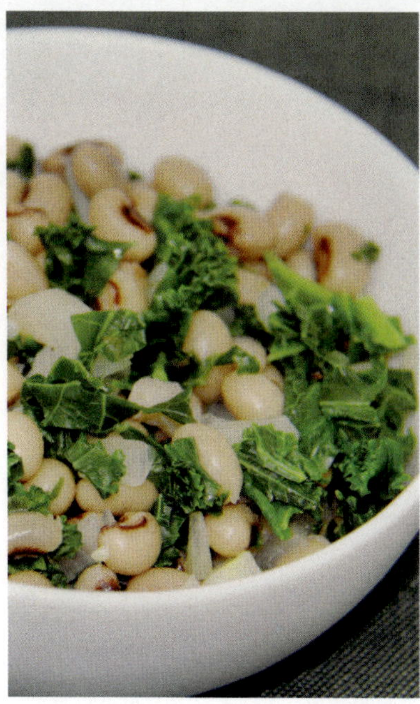

BLACK EYED PEAS WITH MUSTARD GREENS

This super nutritious dish is great as a main course with roasted yellow or sweet potatoes or as a side dish.

1 medium onion, diced (about 1 cup)

2 cups black eyed peas, soaked overnight in water

1 tsp cumin

¼ tsp mustard powder

Black pepper to taste

1 bunch mustard greens, chopped

1 tsp *salt* (gradually reduce or omit)

servings

5–8

1. Water sauté the onions until soft.

2. In a medium pot, add the peas and everything except the mustard greens and salt. Add water to an inch above the peas, and bring to a boil. Simmer for 30–45 minutes.

3. Add the mustard greens and simmer for 5 more minutes. Season to taste with salt, if using.

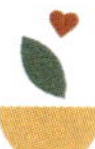

BLACK BEAN AND CORN CHILI

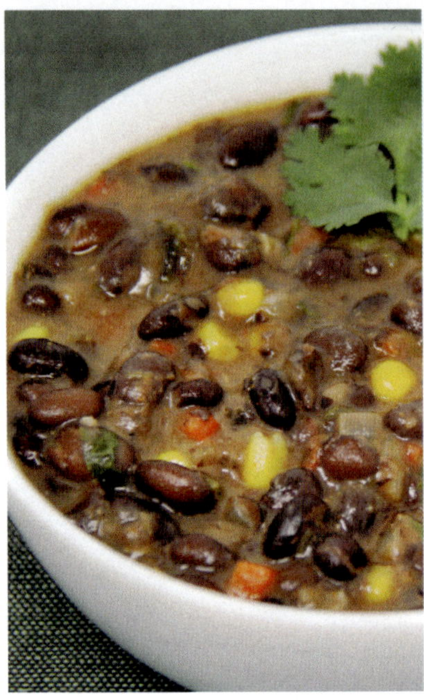

I love serving this hearty chili on Savory Cornbread (p 86) and topping it with Taco Slaw (p 28). Garnish with Salsa (p 101), Sour Cream (p 102), and green onions, and serve with a side of green salad. Keep leftovers in sealed containers in the refrigerator or freezer.

3 poblano peppers

2 cans (15 oz) black beans, preferably low salt, or 3 cups homemade (p 119), drained and mashed

1 large onion, chopped (about 1 ½ cups)

1 red bell pepper, diced

2 tbsp–¼ cup diced jalapeños or to taste

2 large cloves garlic, pressed

3 cans black beans, preferably low salt, or 4½ cups homemade (p 119), rinsed and drained (set aside some of the liquid if desired)

1 cup fresh, frozen and thawed, or canned and drained corn kernels

2 tbsp tomato paste, preferably low salt

2 tsp chili powder or to taste

2 tsp cumin

2 cups water (bean liquid can be included in this)

1 tsp *salt* or to taste (gradually reduce, omit or just add at the table if needed)

½ cup chopped cilantro

servings

6–8

equipment

Immersion blender

1. Broil the poblano peppers until charred. Remove from heat and let sit in a covered container for 10–15 minutes, then peel, seed, and dice.

2. Mash the first quantity of black beans with an immersion blender.

3. In a large skillet, water sauté the onions and red bell pepper until soft. Add the jalapeños and garlic and cook for another minute.

4. Add the whole and mashed beans, poblano peppers, corn, tomato paste, chili powder, cumin, and water. Reduce heat to medium low and simmer for 10 minutes or until it reaches the desired thickness.

5. Stir in salt (optional) and cilantro, cover and let sit a few minutes before serving.

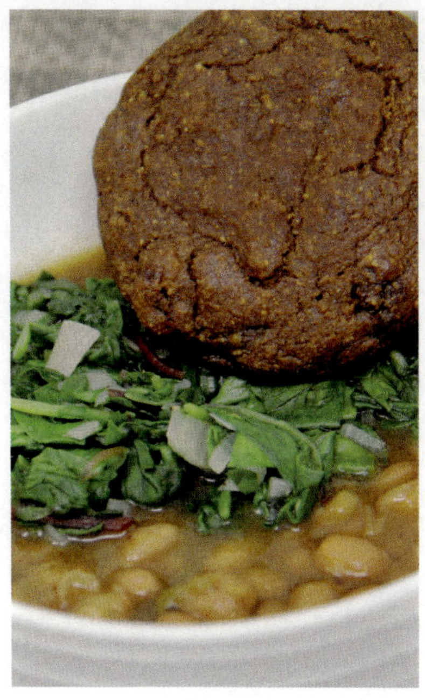

BOSTON STYLE BAKED BEANS

This classic bean dish makes a great side dish for burgers or can be eaten as a main course. Serve with Boston Brown Bread (p 80) and air fried Sweet Potato Fries (p 68). And don't forget to add a scoop of Sautéed Greens (p 76)!

½ cup pitted, chopped medjool dates

1 cup boiling water

1 medium sweet onion, diced (about 1 cup)

1 medium green pepper, diced (about 1 cup)

1 lb dried navy beans or other small white beans, soaked overnight in water

¼ cup *molasses*

2 tsp dry mustard

1 tsp *salt* (gradually reduce or omit)

Black pepper to taste

servings

8–10

equipment

Instant Pot or Crockpot (optional), bullet-style blender

1. In a medium bowl, add the dates and boiling water, cover, and let stand 5 minutes.

2. Water sauté the onions and bell pepper until soft.

3. Rinse the beans, drain, and place in a large pot, Instant Pot or Crockpot.

4. Blend the dates and water in a bullet-style blender.

5. Add all ingredients, including the date mixture, except the salt and pepper to the pot with the beans and mix until combined. Add water to an inch above the beans.

6. On the stovetop, bring mixture to a boil and simmer for 2 hours or until the beans are tender. Cook on high in the crockpot for 8–10 hours or on low for 12–14 hours. Either way, check the beans periodically to make sure there is enough water. Alternatively, place the everything in an Instant Pot and pressure cook for 25 minutes. Add salt (optional) and pepper to taste.

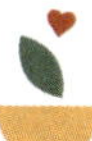

CREAM OF BROCCOLI SOUP

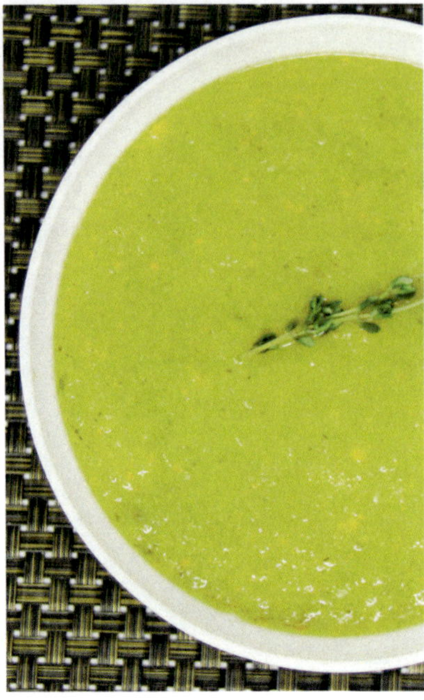

The potatoes make this soup thick and rich without the cream. Enjoy this with Caramelized Onion Naan Bread (p 82) or Green Onion and Jalapeño Cornbread Biscuits (p 83).

1 large onion, chopped (about 1½ cups)

1 carrot, peeled and chopped

3 celery stalks, chopped

4 cups chopped broccoli (cut tops into small florets and chop stems into small pieces, keeping stems separate from florets)

2 medium potatoes, peeled and chopped into 1-inch pieces

6 cups vegetable stock (it's okay to replace some of the vegetable stock with water)

1½ tsp dried thyme, or 2 tbsp minced fresh thyme

½ tsp dried dill, or 2 tsp chopped fresh dill

1 tsp *salt* (gradually reduce or omit)

Black pepper to taste

servings

6–8

equipment

Immersion blender or blender

1. Water sauté the onions, carrots, celery, and broccoli stems until tender.

2. Add the rest of the ingredients, bring to a boil, and simmer for 20–30 minutes.

3. Purée in a blender or with an immersion blender to the desired consistency.

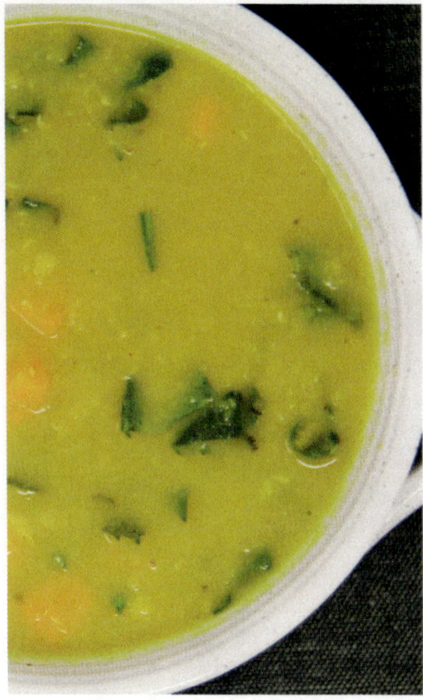

DAL

This hearty and delicious Indian staple dish is a filling meal in itself. I add the baby dark, leafy greens, although including these is less traditional. I like to serve it with Caramelized Onion Naan Bread (p 82) and/or air fried Sweet Potato Fries or French Fries (p 68). You can also garnish it with Sour Cream (p 102) and chopped cilantro.

servings

10–12

equipment

Mortar and pestle (optional)

1 large onion, diced (about 1½ cups)

1 large carrot, diced

2 large garlic cloves, minced

2 jalapeños, cored, seeded, and minced

2 cups dried red lentils

2 tbsp grated fresh ginger

1 tbsp cumin seeds, toasted and crushed in a mortar and pestle or 2 tsp ground cumin

2 tsp yellow curry powder

8 cups vegetable broth, preferably low salt

1 can (15 oz) diced tomatoes, preferably low salt

2 tbsp tomato paste, preferably low salt

2 medium potatoes, diced (about 2½ cups)

2 small sweet potatoes, diced (about 2 cups)

Dash of *maple syrup* (optional)

1 bay leaf

4 cups chopped baby dark, leafy greens (kale, chard, spinach) (optional)

Salt and pepper to taste (eventually omit salt)

1. In a large pot, water sauté the onion and carrots until soft.

2. Add garlic, jalapeño, lentils, ginger, cumin, and curry powder, and sauté for 1–2 minutes or until the herbs and spices are fragrant.

3. Add the vegetable broth, tomatoes, tomato paste, potatoes, sweet potatoes, maple syrup, and bay leaf. Bring to a boil and simmer for 30–45 minutes.

4. Add dark, leafy greens and cook for the last 10 minutes. Add salt (optional) and pepper to taste.

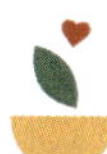

HEARTY MINESTRONE SOUP

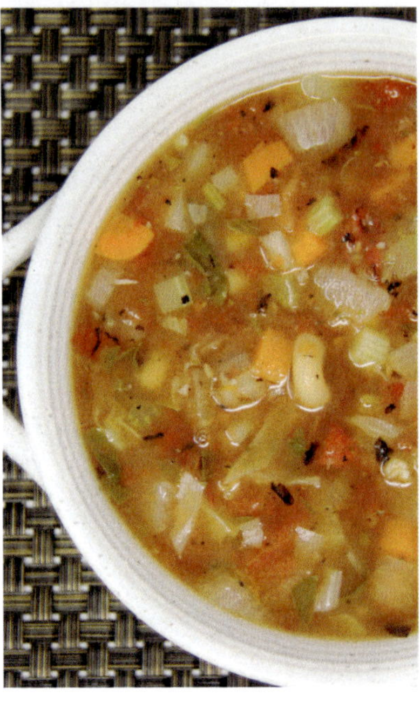

This hearty soup is a complete meal in itself. It is perfect for freezing in sealed containers to take to work or school.

1 medium onion, diced (about 1 cup)

2 medium carrots, diced

2 stalks celery, diced

4 cloves garlic, pressed

1 cup chopped savoy cabbage

2 cans (15 oz) fire roasted tomatoes, preferably low salt

3 cups vegetable broth, preferably low salt

2 cups water

1 can (15 oz) kidney beans, preferably low salt, or 1½ cups homemade (p 119)

1 can (15 oz) navy or cannellini beans, preferably low salt, or 1½ cups homemade (p 119)

2 tbsp red wine vinegar

1½ tbsp Italian seasoning

½–1 cup dried small whole wheat or quinoa pasta shells (optional)

2–4 cups fresh baby spinach or baby dark, leafy greens, roughly chopped

Salt and pepper to taste (eventually omit salt)

servings

8—10

1. Over medium heat, water sauté the onion, carrots, and celery until softened. Add garlic and cook for 1 more minute. Add cabbage and cook until softened.

2. Add tomatoes, vegetable broth, water, beans, vinegar, and Italian seasoning.

3. Cover and bring to boil, then simmer 30 minutes.

4. Add pasta and simmer for 10 more minutes.

5. Remove from heat and stir in baby spinach or dark, leafy greens. Add salt (optional) and pepper to taste.

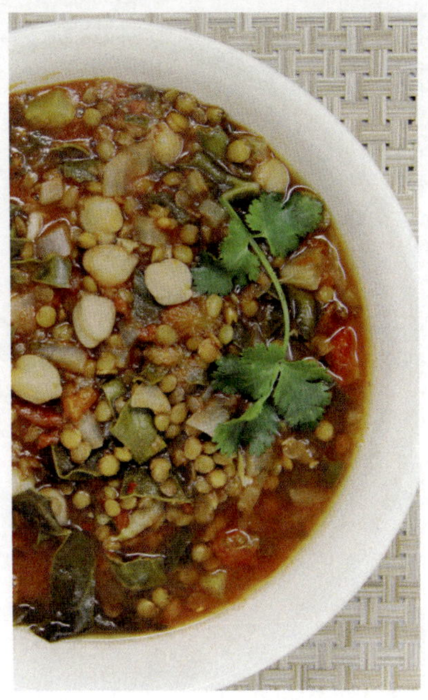

MOROCCAN LENTIL AND GARBANZO BEAN SOUP

This delicious soup is packed with protein, and the hot pepper used to season it (optional) has so many health benefits! I love the tangy flavor of the Swiss chard and lemon juice. Serve with Caramelized Onion Naan Bread (p 82), and garnish with Sour Cream (p 102) and fresh cilantro.

servings

10–12

equipment

Instant Pot or Crockpot (optional), bullet-style blender

1 large onion, diced (about 1½ cups)

2 celery stalks, diced

1 bunch Swiss chard, finely chopped (keep the stems separate from leaves)

5 garlic cloves, pressed

1 tbsp fresh grated ginger

2 tsp ground coriander

1 tsp ground cumin

1 tsp harissa powder (caution, this will be spicy, reduce for a milder flavor)

½ tsp red pepper flakes or to taste

4 cups vegetable broth, preferably low salt

4 cups water

2 cans (15 oz) crushed tomatoes, preferably low salt

1 can (15 oz) garbanzo beans, preferably low salt, or 1½ cups homemade (p 119), rinsed and drained

2 cups dried brown or French lentils

1 tsp *salt* (gradually reduce or omit)

Pepper to taste

½ cup minced fresh cilantro

¼ cup minced fresh parsley

2 tbsp lemon juice

1. Water sauté the onions, celery, and Swiss chard stems until soft. Add garlic and ginger and sauté for 1 minute. Stir in coriander, cumin, harissa, and red pepper flakes and cook for 1 more minute.

2. Add broth, water, tomatoes, garbanzo beans, lentils, and Swiss chard leaves, and bring to a boil.

3. Simmer for about 30 minutes or until the lentils are cooked.

4. Remove from the heat and stir in the cilantro, parsley, and lemon juice. Add salt (optional) and pepper to taste.

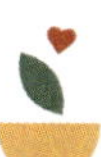

POTATO LEEK SOUP

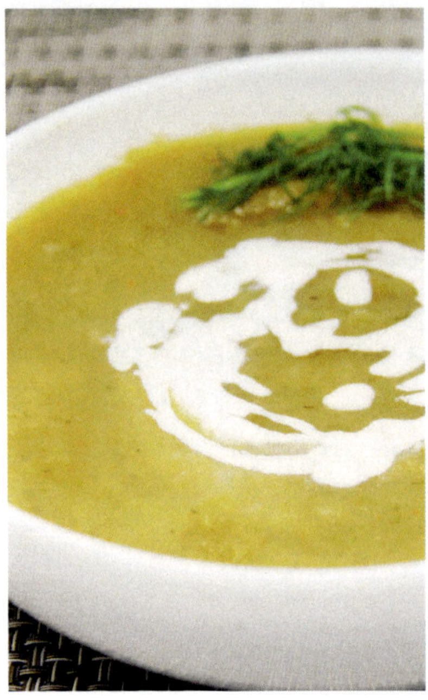

Leeks and potatoes are a powerful combination for both flavor and nutrients. Serve this hearty winter soup garnished with Sour Cream (p 102) and chopped chives.

1 large onion, chopped (about 1 ½ cups)

3 celery stalks, chopped

6–8 medium potatoes, peeled and chopped into 1-inch pieces

2 large leeks, sliced into ¼-inch rounds

6 cups vegetable stock, preferably low salt, or 6 cups water

1½ tsp dried thyme, or 2 tbsp chopped fresh thyme

½ tsp dried dill, or 2 tsp chopped fresh dill

1 tsp *salt* (gradually reduce or omit)

Black pepper to taste

servings

About 6

equipment

Immersion blender or blender

1. Water sauté the onions and celery until tender.

2. Add the rest of the ingredients and cook for 20–30 minutes.

3. Purée in a blender or with an immersion blender.

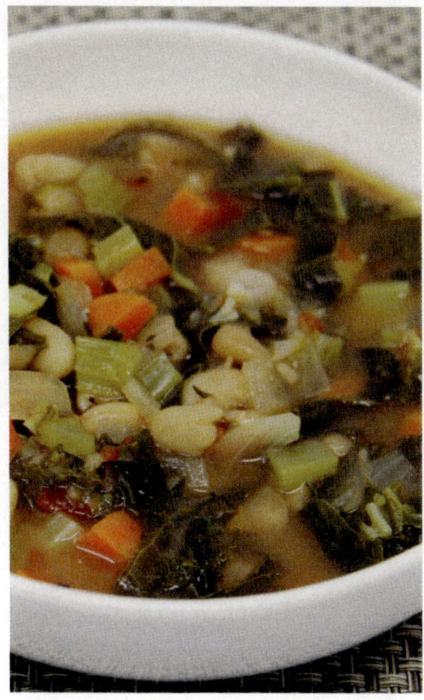

SOUTHWESTERN KALE AND WHITE BEAN SOUP

This is a southwestern twist on a standard Italian favorite. The quinoa boosts the protein and makes it more filling. I love the spicy version with the red pepper flakes and jalapeño. The immersion blended navy beans thicken the soup nicely and the miso adds extra flavor. Enjoy with Green Onion and Jalapeño Cornbread Biscuits (p 83).

Note: for a traditional Kale and White Bean Soup, omit the jalapeños, red pepper flakes, quinoa, and cilantro.

servings

10

equipment

Immersion blender

2 cans (15 oz) navy beans, preferably low salt, or 3 cups homemade (p 119), drained and rinsed

2 tbsp chickpea or soy miso (optional, for extra flavor), preferably low salt

1 large onion, diced (about 1½ cups)

2 medium carrots, diced

2 large celery stalks, diced

3 garlic cloves, pressed

1 jalapeño, minced (optional, if you like spicy)

1½ tbsp dried Italian seasoning

Pinch of red pepper flakes (optional, if you like spicy)

½ cup dried quinoa

2 cans (15 oz) cannellini or great northern beans, preferably low salt, or 3 cups homemade (p 119), drained and rinsed

1 can (15 oz) diced, fire roasted tomatoes with juice, preferably low salt

8 cups vegetable broth, preferably low salt

1 bunch green curly kale, stripped of stems and finely chopped

½ cup coarsely chopped cilantro

Salt and pepper to taste (eventually omit salt)

1. In a medium bowl, mash the navy beans and the miso with an immersion blender and set aside.

2. In a large pot, water sauté onions, carrots, and celery for 5 minutes. Add garlic and jalapeño and cook for another minute.

3. Add the Italian seasoning, pepper flakes, quinoa, whole beans, mashed beans and miso, tomatoes, and vegetable broth or water.

4. Bring to a boil, cover, and simmer for 25 minutes.

5. Add kale and let simmer, stirring occasionally, until kale wilts. Remove from heat and add cilantro.

6. Season to taste with salt (optional) and pepper.

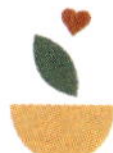

SPLIT PEA AND SWEET POTATO SOUP

This is a hearty winter soup. Try dipping air fried French Fries or Sweet Potato Fries (p 68) in it.

Note: for a more traditional and less sweet soup, reduce or omit the sweet potatoes.

1 large onion, chopped (about 1½ cups)

3 celery stalks, chopped

2 medium carrots, chopped

4 cups vegetable broth, preferably low salt

2 cups water (a little less for thicker soup)

2 cups split peas

½ tsp dried thyme

1 bay leaf

2 cups cubed sweet potato (¼-inch cubes)

Salt and pepper to taste (eventually omit salt)

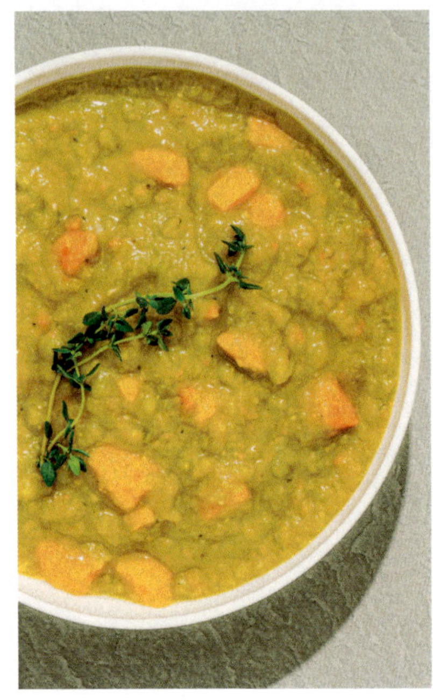

servings

About 6

equipment

Immersion blender

1. In a large pot, water sauté the onion, celery, and carrots until soft.

2. Add vegetable broth, water, split peas, thyme, and bay leaf.

3. Bring to a boil, cover pot, and simmer for 1 hour, stirring occasionally.

4. Remove bay leaf and blend with an immersion blender.

5. Add the sweet potato pieces and cook another 30 minutes or until the sweet potatoes are tender.

6. Season to taste with salt (optional) and pepper.

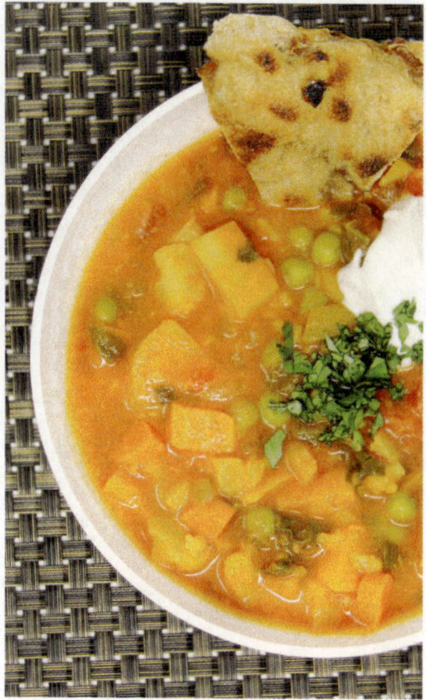

servings

10

VEGETABLE CURRY

This completely from scratch, tomato based curry is delicious topped with Sour Cream (p 102), fresh cilantro, and green onions. Try serving it with Caramelized Onion Naan Bread (p 82). I always make a double batch and freeze it. If you prefer yellow curry, make the Dal (p 43).

1 large onion, diced (about 1½ cups)

4 cloves garlic, pressed

1 jalapeño, seeded and minced

1 tbsp fresh grated ginger

1 tbsp ground coriander

1½ tsp ground cumin

1 tbsp fresh grated turmeric

½ tsp cayenne pepper

1 tbsp tomato paste

2 cups vegetable broth, preferably low salt

1 cup light coconut milk

1 head cauliflower or broccoli, cut into florets

2 medium potatoes, peeled and cubed

2 medium sweet potatoes, peeled and cubed

2 cans (15 oz) crushed tomatoes, preferably low salt

1 cup fresh or frozen peas

1 can (15 oz) garbanzo beas, preferably low salt, or 1½ cups homemade (p 119, optional)

4 cups lightly packed baby spinach

1 whole lime, zested and juiced (about 2 tbsp juice)

Salt and pepper to taste (gradually reduce or omit salt)

1. In a large pot, water sauté the onions until soft. Add garlic, jalapeño, and ginger and cook for 1 minute. Add the remaining spices except salt and pepper and stir for 30 seconds. Stir in the tomato paste.

2. Add the vegetable broth and coconut milk and bring to a boil. Reduce the heat and simmer for 10 minutes.

3. Add the cauliflower or broccoli, potatoes, sweet potatoes, tomatoes, peas, and garbanzo beans, if using, and simmer for 20–25 minutes.

4. Remove from heat and stir in the baby spinach, lime zest, and juice. Season to taste with salt (optional) and pepper.

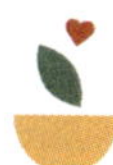

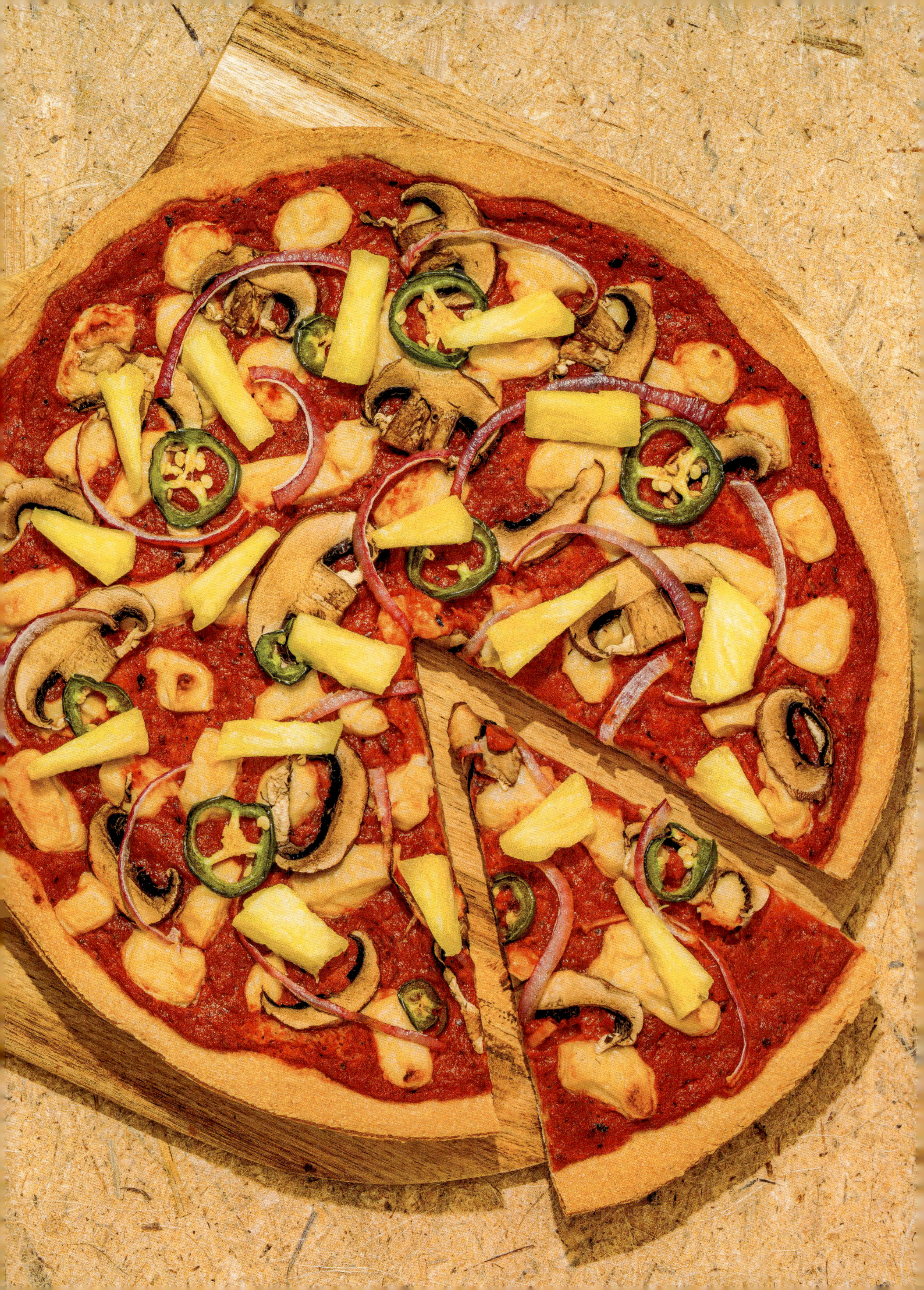

FUN FAVORITES

These recipes are whole food, plant based versions of our favorite comfort foods. I was so happy when I discovered that I would again be able to enjoy my favorite indulgence foods such as pizza, spaghetti, falafel, and more without the consequences. Now I enjoy these foods twice as much because they are nourishing me and keeping me healthy as well as tasting great.

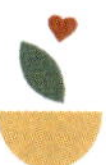

AVOCADO TOAST

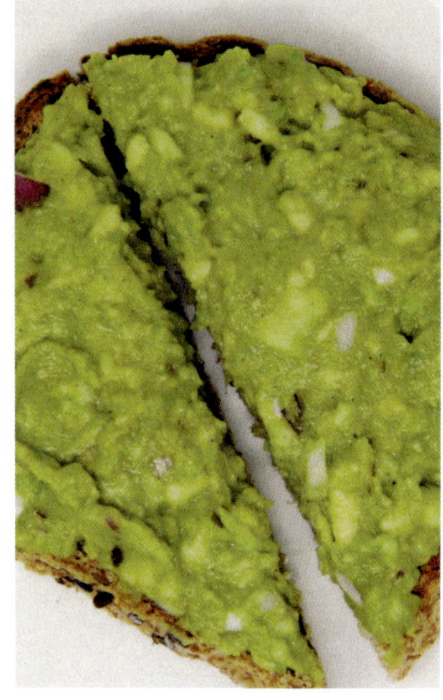

This is a great snack or meal combined with salad or greens. It is also a good thing to order (on whole grain bread) if you are at a restaurant with limited vegan options. Please note that some doctors recommend keeping consumption of nuts and avocados to a minimum on the WFPB food plan, because they are higher in calories and oils, even though they are WFPB and contain beneficial oils.

I often enjoy this made with just avocado slices and seasonings on WFPB toast. You can also add sliced veggies such as onion, tomato, and bell peppers, or make a mashed version like the one below.

servings

2

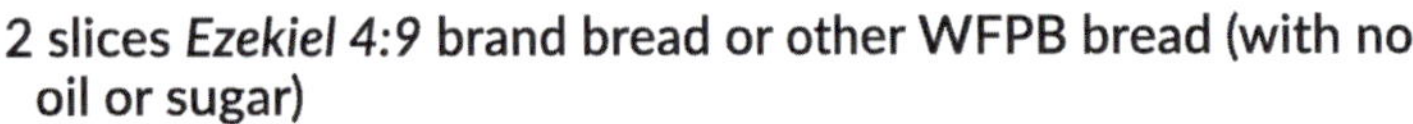

2 slices *Ezekiel 4:9* brand bread or other WFPB bread (with no oil or sugar)

1 large ripe avocado, peeled, pitted, and mashed

2 tbsp finely minced red onion

1 tsp fresh lemon juice

Salt and pepper to taste (eventually omit salt)

1. Toast the bread.

2. With a fork, stir the red onion and lemon juice into the mashed avocado.

3. Spread the mashed avocado mixture on the toast, add seasonings to taste and serve immediately.

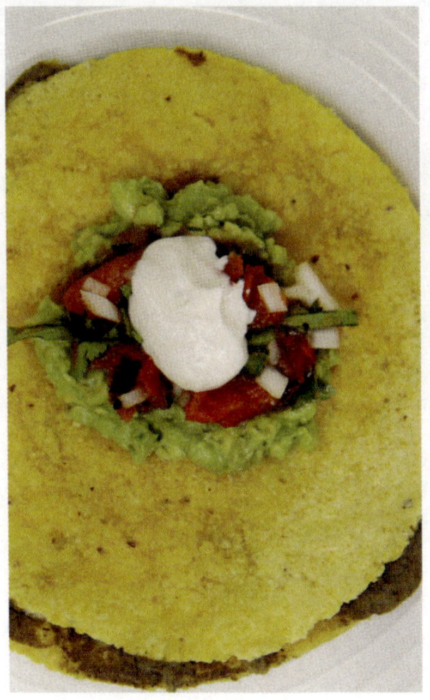

BEAN AND CHEESE QUESADILLAS

These melty quesadillas are satisfying and flavorful. For a more traditional quesadilla, omit the beans and add more cheese. Try adding sautéed mushrooms, tomatoes, onions or jalapeños to the filling to suit your tastes.

1 can (15 oz) black beans, preferably low salt, or 1 ½ cups homemade (p 119, spicy optional), mashed or 1 cup Nacho Bean Dip (p 100)

8 organic sprouted corn tortillas (small, about 6 inches in diameter)

1 cup Nacho Cheese Sauce (p 111)

½ cup diced or thinly sliced sweet or red onion (optional)

1 jalapeño cored, seeded, and minced (optional)

Spray *avocado oil* (eventually omit)

Garnish with any of the following

Sliced avocado or Guacamole (p 95)

Sour Cream (p 102)

Salsa (p 101)

Sliced green onions

Sliced black olives

Note: If you don't have spicy black beans, you can add the following to a can of regular black beans: 1 tsp garlic powder, 1 tsp cumin, ½ tsp chili powder.

servings

4

equipment

Immersion blender, nonstick griddle

1. Preheat a nonstick griddle to 400°F.

2. Rinse and drain the black beans and reserve ¼ cup bean liquid. In a medium bowl, mash the beans and liquid with an immersion blender.

3. Lay the 8 tortillas out on a breadboard or countertop.

4. Spread a layer of mashed beans or Nacho Bean Dip on four of the tortillas. Sprinkle diced onion and diced jalapeño (or other vegetables, if using) on the mashed beans.

5. Spread a layer of Nacho Cheese Sauce on the other four tortillas.

6. Place the tortillas with the cheese sauce face down on the tortillas with beans.

7. Spray the griddle with a thin layer of avocado oil, if using. Place the quesadillas on the griddle and cook for 5 minutes on each side.

8. Garnish and serve immediately.

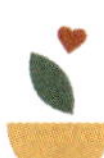

BUTTERNUT SQUASH AND CARAMELIZED ONION PIZZA

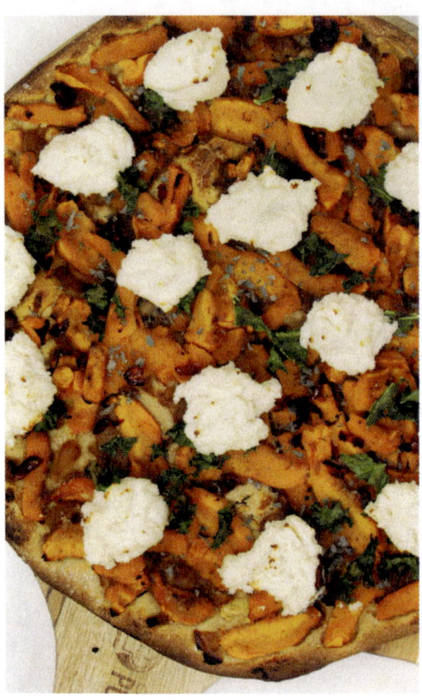

This gourmet pizza has a wonderful blend of flavors. It is a perfect fall or winter dish. Make two and freeze one for later! Make sure to start the pizza dough an hour and a half before you will need to assemble the pizza for baking. If you are only making one pizza, then refrigerate or freeze the other half of the dough for later use.

1 small butternut squash (about 2 lbs whole)

½ cup Caramelized Onions (p 118) (made from about 2 ½ cups diced onions)

1 head garlic

½ batch of Pizza Dough (p 84) or other WFPB pizza base

½ cup chopped kale, stalks removed

1 tbsp chopped fresh sage

1 cup Almond Ricotta Cheese (p 110)

1 tbsp coarsely chopped *dried cranberries* (optional)

Salt to taste (eventually omit)

servings

One 14–16" pizza

equipment

Parchment paper, pizza stone, rolling pin, pizza peel (optional)

1. Preheat the oven to 400°F. Line a baking sheet with parchment paper.

2. Slice the whole squash in half lengthwise and place the two halves with the open side up on the parchment-lined baking sheet. Chop the top off a head of garlic and place it in a garlic roaster or wrap loosely in foil. Place both the squash and garlic in the oven and bake for 30–40 minutes or until the squash is just tender when pricked with a fork. The flesh should still be orange. The garlic should also be soft. Note: if you do not have Caramelized Onions (p 118) already prepared, make them while the squash and garlic are roasting.

3. Remove the squash and garlic from the oven when ready and let cool for a few minutes.

4. Preheat a pizza stone in the oven to 500°F.

5. Carefully slice the rind off the squash and cut it widthwise into slices that are ⅛–¼ inch thick. Set aside.

6. Squeeze the roasted garlic cloves out of their skin into a small bowl, mash with a fork, and set aside.

7. Roll the pizza dough into a circle (14–16 inches in diameter) on a piece of parchment paper, and gently spread the roasted garlic on it with a small spatula. Place the butternut squash slices on the base of the pizza; it is okay for them to overlap. Sprinkle the caramelized onions evenly on top of the butternut squash.

8. Place the pizza, still on the parchment paper, on the pizza stone in the oven and bake for 12 minutes. Remove the pizza from the oven and take off the parchment paper.

9. Sprinkle the kale and sage on top of the pizza. Add dollops of almond ricotta cheese to the top of the pizza so that there is a dollop of ricotta cheese for each of the 8 slices when it is cut. Sprinkle on the cranberries.

10. Bake the pizza directly on the stone for 4–6 more minutes or until some tips on the ricotta cheese are lightly browned. Remove, slice, and serve right away. After slicing the pizza, I like to serve it on the hot pizza stone on a trivet to keep it warm.

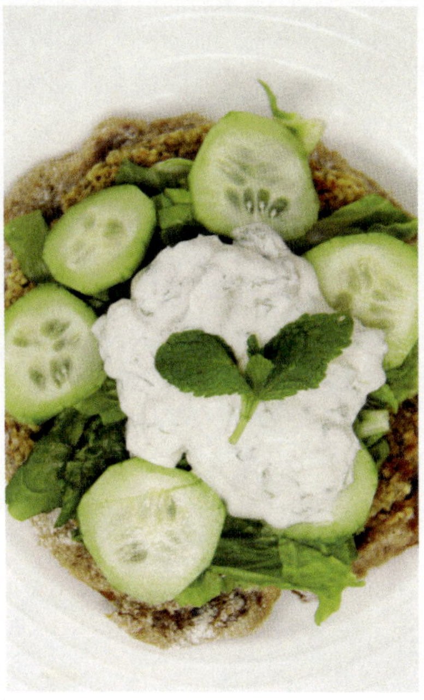

FALAFEL

These are an oil-free version of a Mediterranean classic. I shape the falafel into patties instead of balls so that they fit better on the bread. Try spicing it up with a little cayenne powder or minced jalapeño pepper. Serve on Caramelized Onion Naan Bread (p 82) with sliced, fresh veggies and Tzatziki (p 105).

servings

8–10 falafel patties

equipment

Food processor, nonstick griddle (optional)

2 cups dried garbanzo beans (should be 4 cups when soaked)

1 small onion, quartered

3 medium garlic cloves

¼ cup coarsely chopped fresh parsley

1 tsp ground coriander

2 tsp ground cumin

2 tbsp garbanzo bean flour

2 tsp fresh lemon juice

¼ tsp cayenne powder or 1 tbsp minced jalapeño (optional, if you like spicy)

1 tsp *salt* (gradually reduce or omit)

Black pepper to taste

1. Soak the garbanzo beans overnight. Drain and rinse them thoroughly. *Do not cook them.*

2. Put the 4 cups of garbanzo beans and all of the other ingredients in a food processor. Pulse or run on medium until all of the ingredients are chopped finely but still a little grainy. It should not be a smooth paste like hummus. Then transfer them to a bowl and stir with a fork. The mixture should be able to stick together.

3. Preheat the oven or a nonstick griddle to 375°F. If baking, place parchment paper on large cookie sheets. Roll the mixture into 2-inch balls and then flatten into ½ inch–thick patties. Place the falafel patties in the oven and cook for 10 minutes, then flip and cook for 10 more minutes. Alternatively, you can cook them on a medium heat nonstick griddle for 10 minutes on each side.

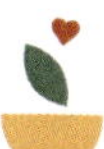

HERBED POLENTA WITH SAUTÉED VEGETABLES

The fresh herbs in this polenta give it a wonderful flavor and boost the nutritional value. You can also serve this polenta in place of whole grain pasta with Spaghetti Sauce (p 61).

4 cups water

1 cup dry polenta

1 tsp *salt* (gradually reduce or omit)

⅓ cup chopped fresh basil

⅓ cup chopped fresh chives

⅓ cup chopped fresh parsley

1. In a medium saucepan, add the water and stir in the dry polenta and salt (optional). Bring to a boil and simmer for 20 minutes with the top on, stirring occasionally.

2. When the polenta is cooked, take the pan off the heat and add the herbs.

Sautéed Vegetables

2 bunches Swiss chard

2 medium shallots, diced (½ cup)

4 garlic cloves, minced

1. Wash the chard and pull the leaves off of the stalks, placing the stalks in a separate pile. Keeping the stalks and leaves separate, chop the stalks finely and the leaves into medium pieces.

2. In a large pan, water sauté the stalks and shallots. When they are tender, add the leaves and garlic and continue sautéing until just tender. Serve on herbed polenta.

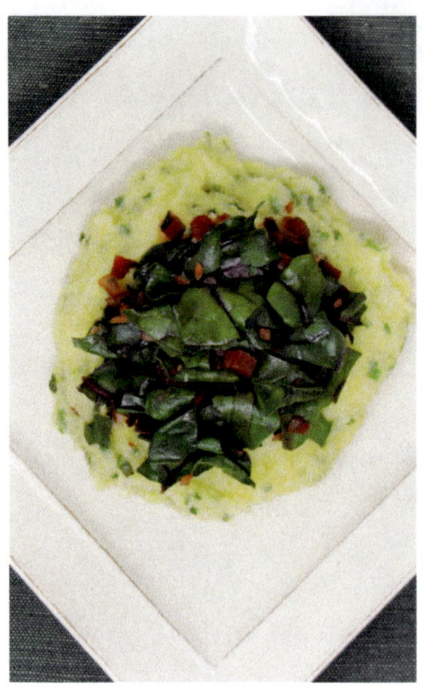

servings

2 large or 4 small

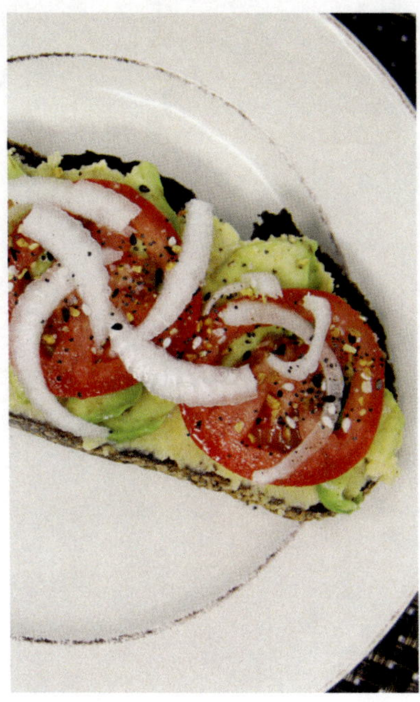

HUMMUS VEGGIE TOAST

This is a great part of a quickie lunch or dinner. Just add a salad or greens and you have a satisfying meal.

Ezekiel 4:9 bread or other whole grain bread (with no oil or sugar)

Hummus (p 96)

Avocado slices

Tomato slices

Raw onion slices

Salt, pepper, and other spices to taste (eventually omit salt)

1. Toast the bread and top with hummus and veggies. Add salt (optional), pepper, and/or other spices to taste.

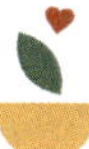

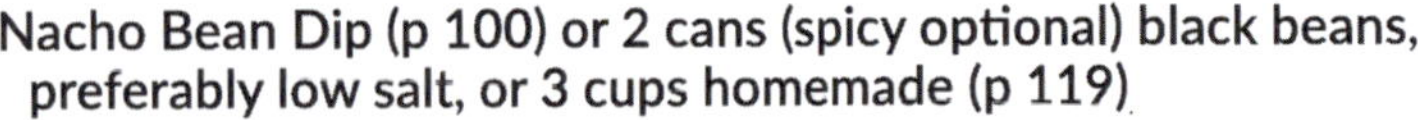

NACHOS

These are a family favorite and come together quickly if you've gotten in the habit of having some of the ingredients on hand. If you don't have anything made already, have family or friends help you, or buy some of the ingredients ready-made, such as the salsa and guacamole. I always serve these with Taco Slaw (p 28) or a green salad. Leftovers can be eaten the next day with chips or on a salad.

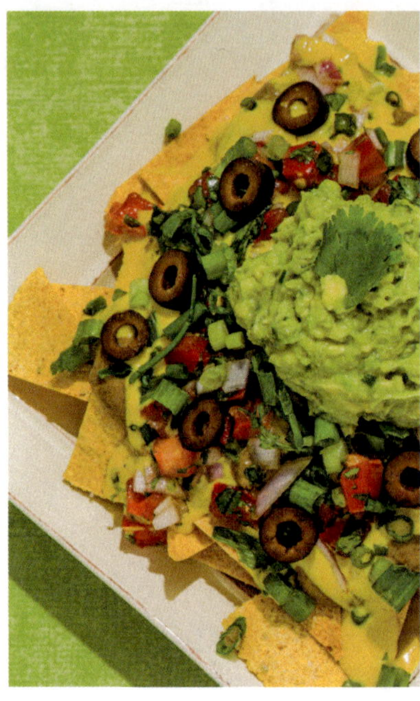

Nacho Bean Dip (p 100) or 2 cans (spicy optional) black beans, preferably low salt, or 3 cups homemade (p 119)

Nacho Cheese Sauce (p 111) or Chipotle Cream (p 91)

Sour Cream (p 102)

Guacamole (p 95)

Salsa (p 101)

1 bunch green onions, sliced

1 small can sliced black olives (optional)

Homemade Tortilla Chips (p 70)

servings

2 large or 4 small

1. Put every ingredient in its own serving bowl.

2. Warm the Beans or Nacho Bean Dip and Nacho Cheese Sauce or Chipotle Cream in the microwave. Do not overheat.

3. If you made the chips in advance, you can place them in a 200°F oven for 5 minutes to warm them just before serving (optional).

4. Place all of the bowls on the table. Pile all of the ingredients on top of the chips, or make a pile of the ingredients on a plate and dip the chips in it.

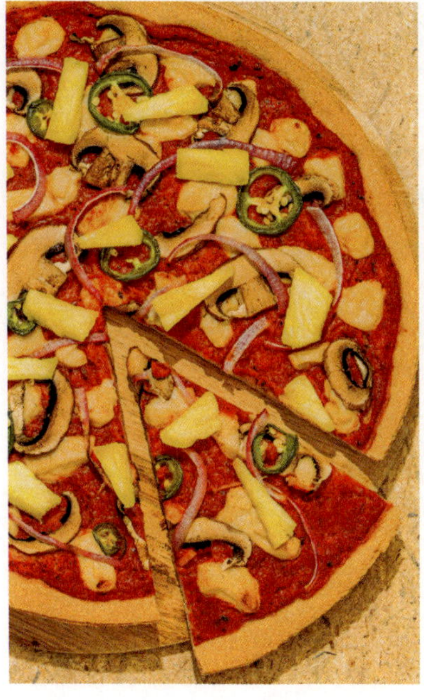

PIZZA

Pizza is something I was really sad to give up when I started to eat WFPB, so I was delighted when I developed a recipe that allowed me to once again enjoy this old favorite. You will be amazed at the crisp crust and melty cheese. I usually make two pizzas and freeze one (after baking) or make two different kinds of pizza and freeze the leftovers. The coarse salt and pepper on the bottom of the crust add a wonderful and unexpected flavor. Try your own combinations. Enjoy!

Note: If you do not already have frozen pizza dough thawed, Make the Pizza Dough (p 84) according to instructions 1½ hours in advance of when you want to assemble the pizza.

servings

One 14–16" pizza

equipment

Pizza stone, rolling pin, parchment paper, pizza peel (optional)

½ batch of Pizza Dough (p 84) or other WFPB pizza base

¾ cup Mozzarella (p 114)

1 cup Pizza Sauce (p 120) or 1 jar (15 oz) pizza sauce, no sugar and preferably low salt and low or no oil

Coarsely ground *salt* and pepper (eventually eliminate salt)

Red pepper flakes, to taste

Veggie Pizza

1 cup sliced crimini mushrooms

1 bell pepper, sliced

1 small red onion, sliced

1 small can sliced black olives

Pizza Margherita

2 fresh tomatoes, sliced (Roma tomatoes are traditionally used)

1 cup fresh basil, chopped

2 cloves garlic, pressed

Lovejoy Combo

1 cup sliced crimini mushrooms

1 cup diced fresh pineapple

1 jalapeño, minced

½ cup sliced red onion

1. Preheat pizza stone(s) in a 500°F oven.

2. Use a rolling pin to roll out the pizza dough into a 14 to 16-inch diameter circle on parchment paper.

3. If you want to add salt and pepper to the bottom of the crust, sprinkle coarse salt and pepper over the circle of dough. Place a piece of parchment on top and gently press or roll the salt and pepper into the dough. Flip the dough with the parchment paper on it, so the salt and pepper side is on the bottom. Remove the top piece of parchment paper.

4. If you are making the Margherita pizza, sprinkle the pressed garlic on the crust.

5. For all variations, spread the pizza sauce on the pizza dough.

6. Spread small pieces of mozzarella evenly over the pizza, then add toppings of your choice.

7. Using a pizza peel or flat baking sheet, move the pizza, keeping the bottom piece of parchment paper attached, onto the pizza stone and bake for 15 minutes.

8. Open the oven and gently lift the pizza off the parchment paper, put it directly on the pizza stone and cook for 5–6 more minutes.

9. Remove pizza from the oven and slice on a cutting board. The pizza can be placed back on the pizza stone on a trivet to keep warm while serving. Don't forget the salad and red pepper flakes!

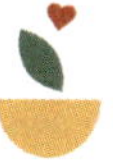

MUSHROOM AND BELL PEPPER GYROS

These are a delicious, high protein, Middle Eastern style meal. I always keep Caramelized Onion Naan Bread (p 82) in the freezer and defrost them whenever I make these.

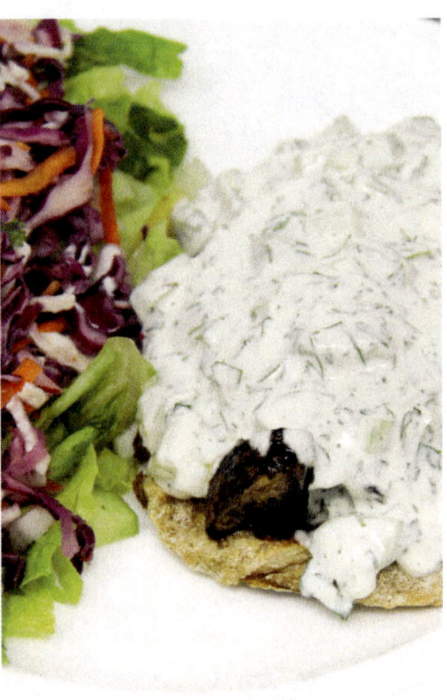

4 Portobello mushroom caps, sliced into ½ inch–wide strips and then into 1½-inch pieces

1 red, yellow, or orange pepper sliced into ¼ inch–wide strips and then 1½-inch pieces

4 tbsp Worcestershire Sauce (p 106) or store bought without anchovies

2 tsp cumin

2 tsp *maple syrup*

1 cup Tzatziki (p 105)

4 medium Caramelized Onion Naan Breads (p 82)

servings

4

1. Place the sliced Portobellos and bell pepper in a glass storage container with a lid.

2. In a small bowl, whisk together the Worcestershire Sauce, cumin, and maple syrup.

3. Pour the Worcestershire Sauce mixture over the mushroom and bell pepper slices, cover tightly, and shake it up. Set aside for 15 minutes.

4. Over medium heat, water sauté the mushrooms and peppers for 4–5 minutes or until tender. Stir often and add small amounts of water to prevent sticking. Remove from heat and let cool for 2–3 minutes.

5. Warm 4 Caramelized Onion Naan Breads in the microwave and/or toaster, top each with the mushroom and pepper mixture, and drizzle with ¼ cup Tzatziki. Serve right away with salad or other greens.

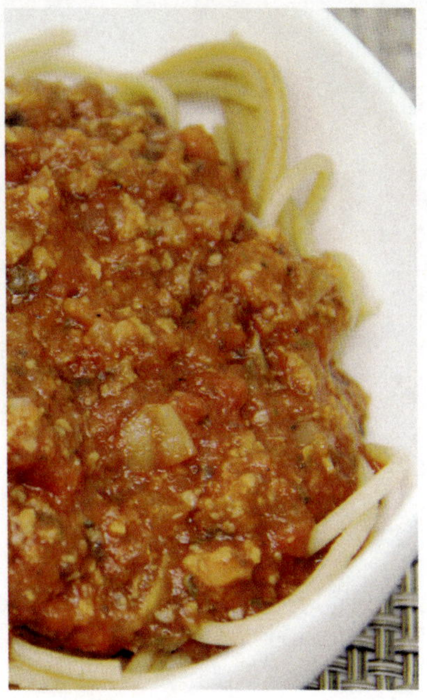

servings

4-6

The olives and pepperoncini give this dish a savory and spicy flavor. The minced mushrooms and tempeh (optional) give the sauce a meatier texture. Serve over whole wheat spaghetti noodles or on Herbed Polenta (p 56) with Roasted Garlic Bread (p 75) and salad.

Please note that the olives and pepperoncini contain salt.

1 small onion, chopped (about ½ cup)

2 medium shallots, finely chopped (about ½ cup)

4 cloves garlic, pressed

2 cans (30 oz) of crushed tomatoes, preferably low salt

2 tbsp tomato paste, preferably low salt

1 tbsp Italian seasoning

1 cup chopped fresh basil

½ cup sliced pepperoncini (optional, for spicy flavor)

½ cup sliced green or kalamata olives (or some of each)

¼ cup pepperoncini water (optional, for spicy flavor)

4 oz tempeh, finely chopped (optional, for texture and added protein)

1½ cups (8 oz) crimini mushrooms, minced

Pepper to taste

2 cups chopped baby dark, leafy greens or baby spinach (optional)

1. Water sauté the onions and shallots until soft. Add the garlic and sauté for 30 more seconds.

2. Add the remaining ingredients except for greens and bring to a boil. Reduce heat and simmer for 15 minutes.

3. Add greens and simmer for 5 more minutes or until the sauce is the desired thickness.

4. Serve with whole grain spaghetti cooked according to instructions on the package or herbed polenta.

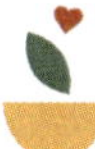

VEGGIE BURGERS

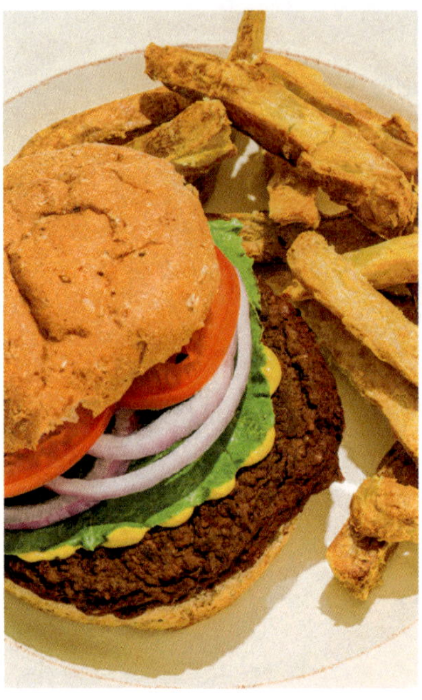

These burgers are packed with healthy ingredients. I like to serve them either on store bought WFPB hamburger buns (*Ezekiel 4:9*, *Engine 2*, or *Alvarado Street Bakery*) or my Caramelized Onion Burger Buns (p 81) with lettuce, pickles, tomato, onion, mustard, and Special Sauce for Veggie Burgers (p 103). The air fried French Fries or Sweet Potato Fries (p 68) are a perfect complement, along with salad and/or fruit.

It's best to cook all of the burgers at once and freeze them for reheating in the microwave or on a griddle.

¼ cup diced shallots

¾ cup diced onions

2 cups sliced crimini mushrooms

1 large clove garlic, pressed

1 cup cooked lentils

1 can black beans, preferably low salt, or 1 ½ cups homemade (p 119), rinsed and drained

1 cup cooked brown rice

½ cup rolled oats

1 tbsp nutritional yeast

2 tbsp Worcestershire Sauce (p 106)

1 tsp *salt* (gradually reduce or omit)

Pepper to taste

servings

About 8

equipment

Nonstick griddle

1. Water sauté the shallots and onions for 5 minutes, add the chopped mushrooms, and cook for 3 more minutes, then add the pressed garlic and cook for 1 more minute.

2. Preheat a nonstick griddle to 350°F.

3. Add all of the ingredients to a food processor and blend until it is a coarse meal.

4. The mixture will be fairly soft, so you will need to use a large spoon to drop the mixture onto the griddle and shape into ½ inch-thick patties with a spatula. Cook for 20 minutes on each side. To make them a little firmer, leave them on the griddle for 15 minutes after you have turned it off.

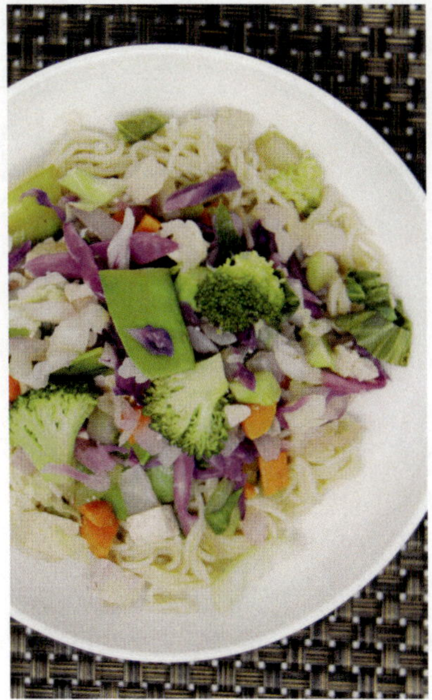

servings

About 6

VEGGIE STIR FRY

I did not think I would ever eat a stir fry again when I gave up oil. However, when I mastered the skill of water sautéing, I was able to once again enjoy one of my favorite meals. Serve with tamari, Korean Style Hot Sauce (p 98), or Indonesian Peanut Sauce (p 97) over brown rice ramen noodles, brown rice, or quinoa. I like to make a big batch and freeze noodles with vegetables in single servings.

¼–½ cup tamari

1½ tsp fresh grated ginger

2 cloves garlic, pressed

1 tbsp fresh lime juice

1 package (16 oz) firm tofu, cut into ¼-inch cubes

1 large onion, chopped (about 1 ½ cups)

1 cup chopped broccoli

1 cup chopped cauliflower

2 celery stalks, chopped

1 carrot, chopped

1 cup sliced green cabbage

1 cup sliced red cabbage

1 cup snow peas, ends removed and cut in half

1 cup sugar snap peas, strings removed and cut into 1-inch pieces

1 cup chopped baby bok choy

4 blocks brown rice and quinoa ramen noodles (10–12 oz)

1. In a glass container with a lid, combine the tamari, grated ginger, garlic, and lime juice. Add the tofu, snap on the lid and shake gently until mixed. Leave the tofu marinating for half an hour or longer.

2. Put 2 quarts of water in a medium pot and place on a stove burner. Do not turn the heat on yet.

3. In a very large pan, water sauté the onions, broccoli, cauliflower, celery, and carrots for 5 minutes. Then add the cabbage, snow peas, snap peas, and bok choy, and cook for another 4 minutes.

4. Turn the burner under the pot of water on high.

5. Add the tofu and the marinade to the vegetables and cook for another 2 minutes. Remove from the heat and cover tightly until the noodles are ready.

6. When the pot of water is boiling, drop in the blocks of ramen noodles. After 1 minute, use two forks to gently pull apart the noodles, then cook for about 3 more minutes. When the noodles are cooked to taste, drain and serve with the stir-fried vegetables and sauce of your choice.

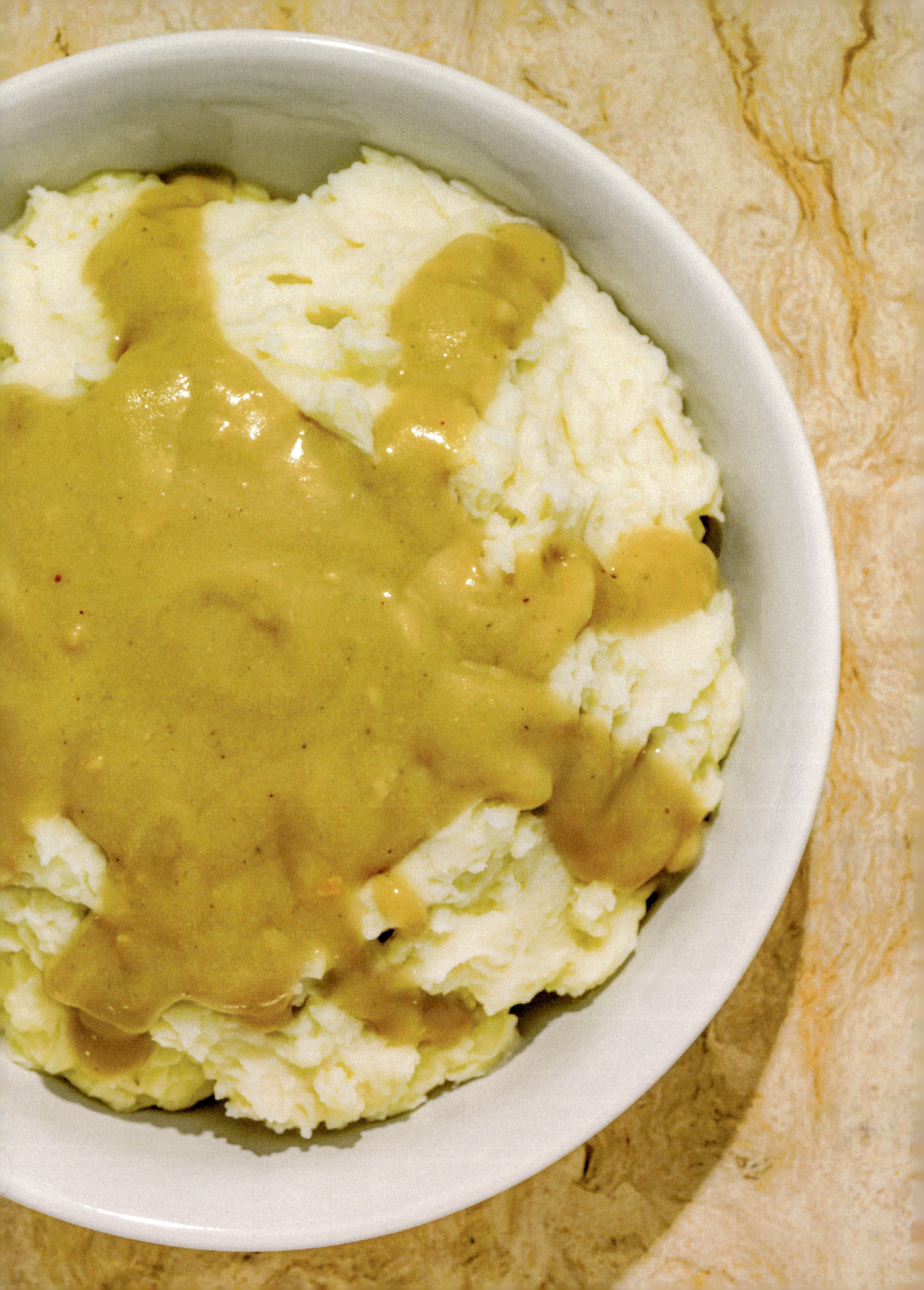

SIDE DISHES

After reading *The Starch Solution* by John McDougall, MD, I have gained a new appreciation for the importance of starch in our diet. Potatoes, sweet potatoes, whole grain breads, brown rice, corn, and legumes are all great fuel for our bodies. I regularly enjoy these healthy versions of baked potatoes with sour cream and green onions, mashed potatoes with stuffing and gravy, french fries, and homemade tortilla chips. Once you transition to these, you too will enjoy both the food and how good you feel after you eat it!

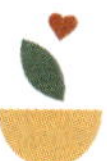

BAKED POTATOES: WHITE OR SWEET

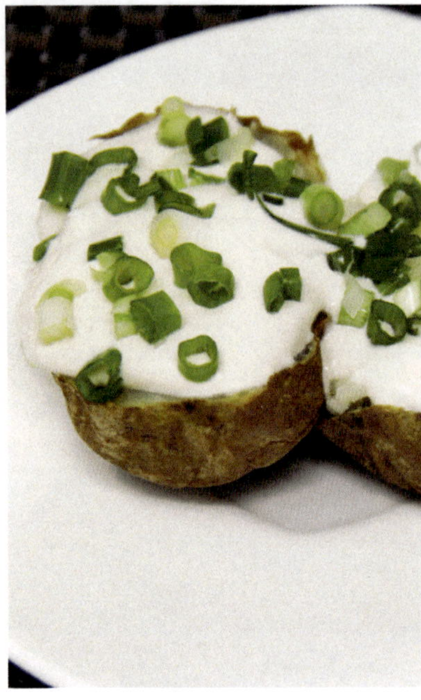

In addition to being delicious, potatoes contain a broad range of nutrients. Top them with Gravy (p 94), chili, baked beans, or sautéed mushrooms and/or Sour Cream (p 102) and green onions.

4 medium potatoes (russet or sweet), washed and scrubbed with a vegetable brush

servings

4

1. Preheat the oven to 375°F.

2. Pierce the potatoes a few times with a knife or fork.

3. Place russet potatoes directly on the baking rack and bake the for 30–40 minutes or until tender all the way through when pierced with a fork or knife.

4. Place sweet potatoes on a baking tray lined with parchment paper and bake for 40–50 minutes or until tender all the way through when pierced with a fork or knife.

Note: if you want to shorten the baking time, microwave each potato for 2 minutes before putting in the oven.

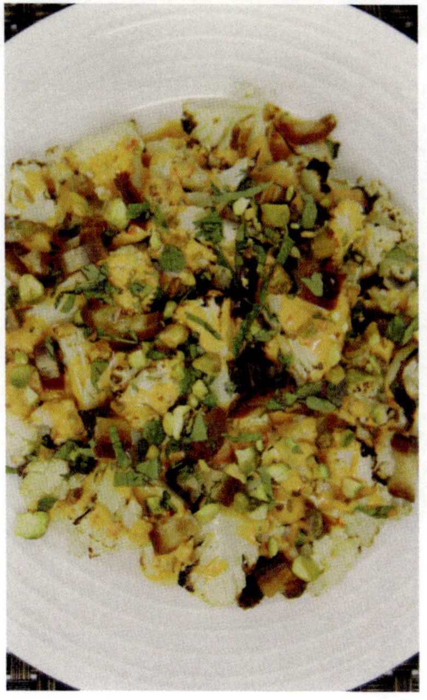

BRAISED CAULIFLOWER WITH HARISSA SAUCE

This makes a wonderful appetizer or side dish. The herbs, dates, and pistachios give it a delightful blend of flavors and textures to complement the spicy harissa sauce.

servings

4

equipment

Bullet-style blender

1 large head of cauliflower cut into bite size florets

2 medium cloves garlic, pressed

¼ cup aquafaba

⅓ cup pitted, diced medjool dates

2 tbsp chopped mint

2 tbsp chopped dill

¼ cup coarsely chopped, toasted pistachios

Harissa Sauce

¼ cup tahini

1 pitted medjool date, chopped

¼ cup boiling water

2 tbsp Soaked Cashews (p 121)

1 medium clove garlic

1 tsp lemon juice

1 tbsp harissa paste or to taste

¼ cup water

½ tsp *salt* (gradually reduce)

1. In a large bowl, whip the aquafaba until stiff. Mix in the pressed garlic and add the cauliflower florets. Stir the florets until they are all coated with the garlic mixture. Let sit at least 20 minutes.

2. Preheat the oven to 500°F and line a baking sheet with parchment paper.

3. Spread the cauliflower florets evenly on the parchment-lined baking sheet.

4. Bake the cauliflower for 15–20 minutes or until lightly browned and tender when pricked with a knife.

5. While the cauliflower is cooking, add the date and boiling water to a small bowl, cover, and let stand 5 minutes. Add all of the Harissa Sauce ingredients, including the date mixture to a bullet-style blender and blend. Add additional water by the tablespoonful to achieve desired consistency.

6. When the cauliflower is ready, remove it from the oven and place it in a medium size serving dish. Drizzle about half of the harissa sauce on the cauliflower and top with diced dates, chopped mint, dill and pistachios.

7. Serve immediately. Freeze or refrigerate the remaining sauce for next time.

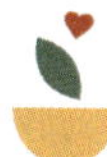

FRENCH OR SWEET POTATO FRIES

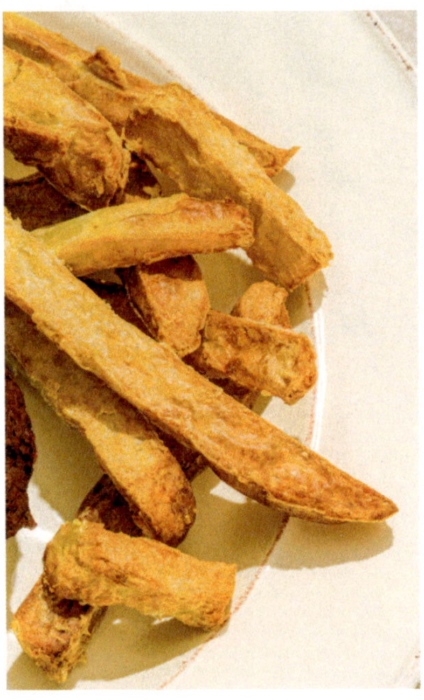

I was so happy when I discovered how to make these delicious air fried French fries and sweet potato fries. Dr. McDougall's book, *The Starch Solution*, inspired me to add more starchy vegetables to my diet. Since I made this change, I have found myself much more satisfied after meals, and my cravings for sweeter foods have almost completely gone away. I used to peel the potatoes, but when I found out how many nutrients we throw away when we don't eat the skins, I stopped peeling them. And they are just as delicious. You will need an air fryer to make these. Go ahead—indulge and enjoy this guilt-free version of an old favorite!

4 russet, yellow, or sweet potatoes, (peeling is optional) sliced into fries (whatever size you like)

5 cups water

2 tbsp baking soda

Your favorite herb or spice mixture, optional

servings

2–4

equipment

Air fryer

1. Cut the potatoes into the desired French fry size and shape.

2. In a medium pot, add the water and baking soda and bring to a boil. For russet or yellow potatoes: when the water is boiling, put the potatoes in and boil for 6 minutes for thick fries or 3 minutes for thin fries. For sweet potatoes: put thick ones in the boiling water for 4 minutes and thin slices in for 2 minutes. Drain the potatoes in a colander.

3. Place the potatoes in an air fryer, and cook according to the air fryer instructions.

4. Remove the potatoes when they are golden brown on the outside. Sprinkle a spice and herb mixture of your choice on the fries and/or dip in mustard, beans, split pea soup, or vinegar.

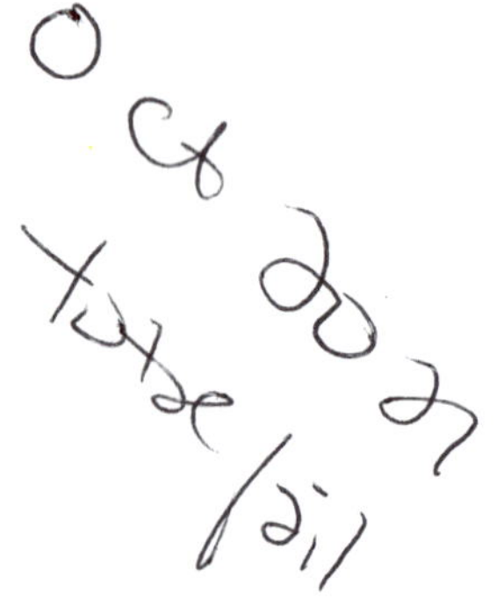

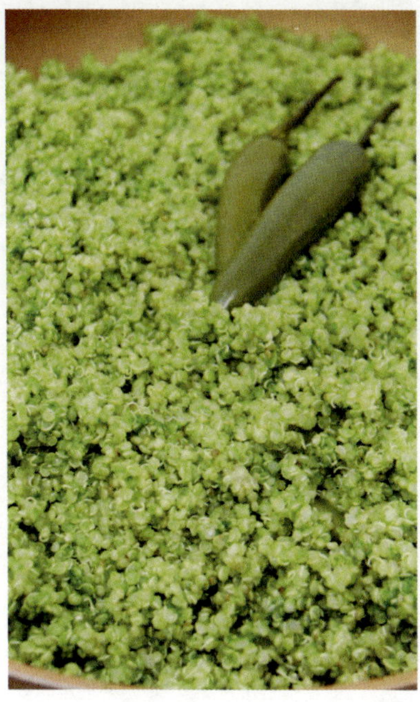

GREEN QUINOA

This is one of my absolute favorite side dishes. It goes very well with all of the southwestern style dishes. Make a large batch and freeze the extra for a flavorful addition to any bowl.

2 cups uncooked quinoa

3 cups water

⅓ cup coarsely chopped white onion

1 small garlic clove

1 tsp *salt* (gradually reduce)

2 whole serrano or jalapeño peppers

servings

6–8

equipment

Bullet-style blender

1. Soak the quinoa for 2 minutes, then rinse and drain in a large sieve. Let it sit in the sieve for another 5 minutes to drain as much water as possible.

2. Meanwhile, combine the water, onion, garlic and salt in a blender and blend until smooth.

3. In a large saucepan, cook the quinoa, stirring constantly until it starts to crackle and becomes dry.

4. Stir the liquid onion mixture into the quinoa and add the whole peppers.

5. Bring to a boil, turn heat to low, cover pan tightly, and simmer for 15–20 minutes, stirring once or twice.

6. While the quinoa is cooking, make the green sauce (see below).

7. Check the quinoa to see whether all the water has been absorbed and the quinoa is completely cooked. When it's done, take off the heat and let it sit for about 5 minutes with the cover on.

8. Stir about half of the green sauce—a little at a time—into the quinoa until it is evenly distributed and has the desired color and taste. Freeze any leftover green sauce.

Green Sauce

3 cups baby spinach, packed

½ cup water

⅓ cup chopped fresh cilantro, packed

1 jalapeño, seeded and coarsely chopped

2 cloves garlic

1 tsp *salt* (gradually reduce)

1. Put the spinach and ¼ cup water into a small saucepan. Cook on medium heat, stirring until the spinach is just wilted and still bright green. Let cool.

2. Pour the spinach and water into a bullet-style blender. Add the cilantro, jalapeño, garlic and salt, and blend until smooth. Add the remaining ¼ cup water if needed to make the mixture wet enough to blend.

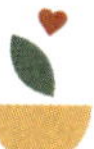

HOMEMADE TORTILLA CHIPS

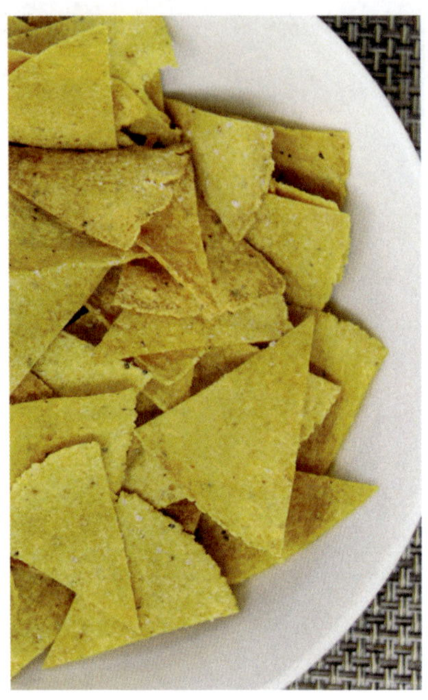

I have tried this recipe with a number of different types of corn tortillas and found it works best with the sprouted corn tortillas from *Food for Life*—and there is some evidence that sprouted grains are even more nutritious than unsprouted. Many of the *Food for Life* products, including their *Ezekiel 4:9* brand bread, use sprouted grains.

1 package organic, sprouted corn tortillas

Water in a spray bottle

Salt (gradually reduce) and/or use other herbs and spices to taste

servings

2–4

equipment

Spray bottle

1. Preheat the oven to 400°F.

2. Cut the stack of tortillas into eighths and lay the triangles out on two large baking sheets. Use a clean spray bottle (I keep a small one in the kitchen for this purpose) to spray the tortilla pieces lightly with water, then sprinkle with a little salt and/or herbs and spices to your taste.

3. Bake the tortilla pieces for 10 minutes or until just starting to brown. Do not remove them too soon or they will be chewy. If not all of them are ready, remove the cooked ones and put the rest back in the oven to bake a minute or two longer. Remove from oven and place in a bowl.

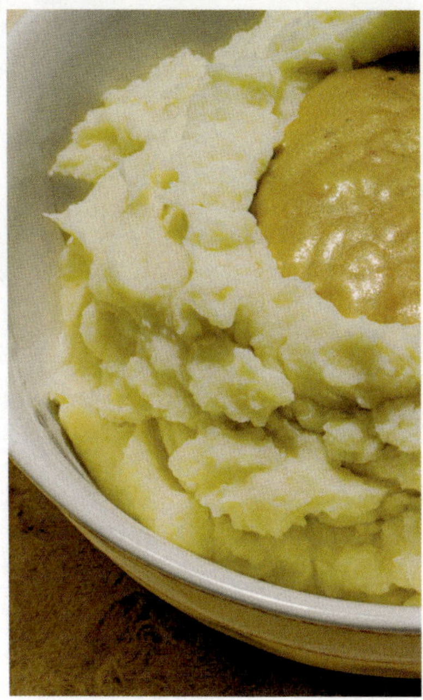

MASHED POTATOES

These are delicious on their own or with Stuffing (p 77) and/or Gravy (p 94). Try adding chopped sweet onion for a change. I also like to take a bowl of mashed potatoes with corn kernels, peas, and broccoli to work as a quick and satisfying lunch.

3 lbs potatoes, peeled and cut into chunks (russet or Yukon gold)

½ cup unsweetened soy or other non-dairy milk

Salt and pepper to taste (eventually omit salt)

1. In a large pot with enough water to cover them, bring the potatoes to a boil and then simmer for around 15 minutes or until they are tender when pierced with a fork or sharp knife. Do not over boil as they will disintegrate and become watery. Drain in a colander.

2. Pour the potatoes back into the pot, add the non-dairy milk, salt, if using, and pepper and either mix with a hand mixer or smash with a potato masher. Add more non-dairy milk for moister potatoes.

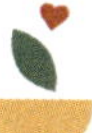

POTATO PANCAKES

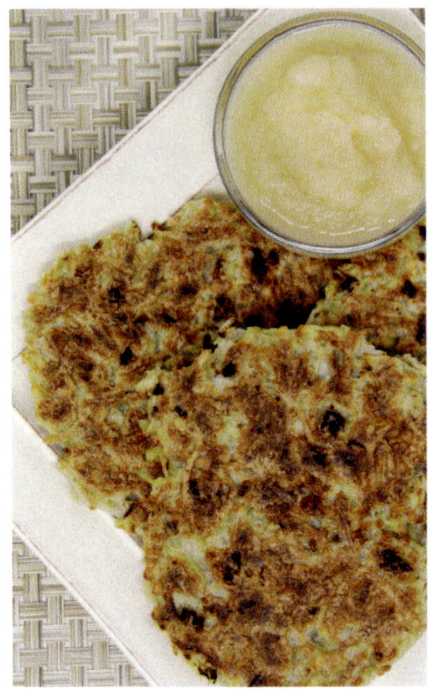

It's great to be able to eat potato pancakes on this food plan. I like to make a double batch and freeze the leftovers. Serve with Apple Sauce (p 90), Sour Cream (p 102), and green onions.

4 cups grated russet or yellow potatoes

1 cup diced onion

⅓ cup aquafaba (use ½ cup for thinner, crisper pancakes)

2 tbsp *potato flour*

1 tsp *salt* (gradually reduce or omit and add at the table if needed)

servings

About 10 pancakes

equipment

Nonstick griddle (optional)

1. Preheat a nonstick griddle to 400°F.

2. In a large bowl, mix the grated potatoes and diced onion.

3. In a small bowl, mix together the potato flour and salt.

4. Add the potato flour and salt to the potatoes and onions and mix well.

5. In a medium bowl, whip the aquafaba until it forms stiff peaks.

6. Fold the whipped aquafaba into the potato mixture.

7. Drop large spoonfuls of the mixture onto the nonstick griddle and shape into round patties with a spatula. Cook for 10–15 minutes on each side or until golden brown.

Note: if you do not have a nonstick griddle, line a baking sheet with parchment paper and bake the pancakes at 425°F for 25 minutes. Flip them at 12 minutes. The pancakes should be golden brown when done.

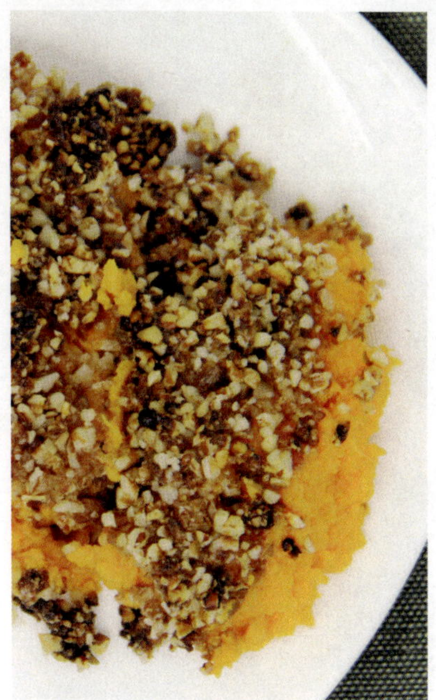

PECAN ENCRUSTED SWEET POTATO PURÉE

The crunchy, chewy texture of the pecans and dates, the luscious color of the potatoes, and the natural sweetness make this a perfect accompaniment to Mashed Potatoes (p 71), Gravy (p 94), and Stuffing (p 77). They are always on my holiday dinner table.

3 lbs sweet potatoes, peeled and cut into chunks

⅓ cup pitted and chopped medjool dates

⅔ cup raw pecans, coarsely chopped

servings

6-8

equipment

Hand mixer, food processor

1. In a large pot, bring the sweet potatoes to a boil and then simmer for around 15 minutes or until they are tender when pierced with a fork or sharp knife. Do not over boil or they will disintegrate and be watery.

2. Preheat the oven to 400°F.

3. When cooked, pour the sweet potatoes into a colander and drain. Then pour them back into the pot or a bowl and mix with a hand mixer until light and fluffy. Transfer the whipped sweet potatoes into a 9" x 7" oval casserole dish.

4. In a small food processor, process the dates and pecans until they are medium ground. Sprinkle the pecan mixture on top of the sweet potatoes.

5. Bake for 30-40 minutes or until the topping is golden brown and crisp.

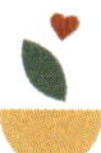

ROASTED ASPARAGUS

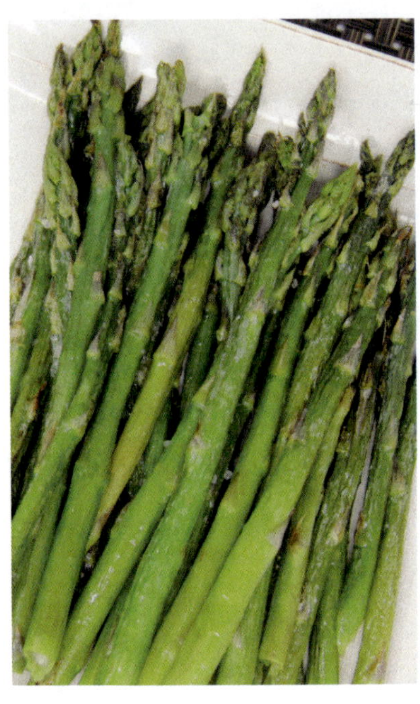

This is my favorite way to cook asparagus. In this instance, using a tiny amount of oil allows you to enjoy a classic, nutritious, and tasty dish.

1 bunch asparagus

Spray *avocado oil*

Salt (gradually reduce)

servings

4

1. Preheat the oven to broil.

2. Snap the bottoms off the asparagus where they naturally break (you may be surprised how much comes off, but that part will be tough, so discard it) and wash them. Lay them out on a baking tray in a single layer. Spray the asparagus lightly with the avocado oil and sprinkle with a little salt.

3. Broil on the highest rack in the oven for approximately 5 minutes or until the asparagus are tender when pricked with a knife. They should not look charred. Serve right away.

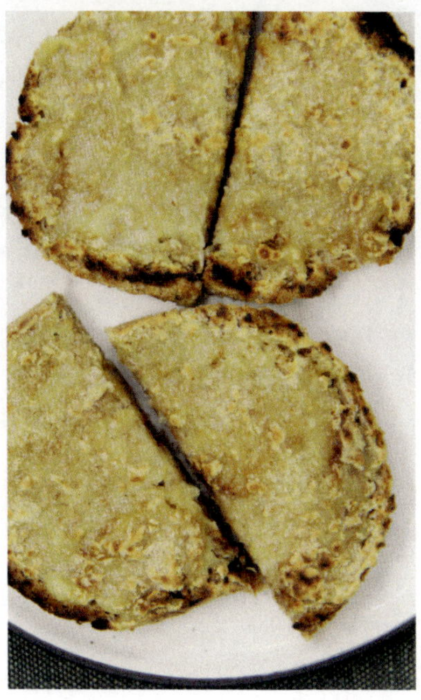

servings

2–4

ROASTED GARLIC BREAD

Garlic is said to have many immune boosting and anticancer properties, and this is a great way to get a big helping of it. This healthy version is a nice alternative to garlic bread that is made with butter or oil. I like to serve it with Spaghetti (p 61) along with a salad or Sautéed Greens (p 76).

2 English muffins or burger buns, or 4 slices of bread (*Ezekiel 4:9* brand bread or other WFPB version)

2 large heads of garlic

Salt and pepper to taste (eventually omit salt)

1. Preheat the oven to 400°F.

2. Cut the tops off of the heads of garlic and place them in a garlic roaster or other covered, oven-safe dish (loosely wrapped aluminum foil can be used, too).

3. Roast the garlic for 40 minutes and check it. It is ready when it is soft all the way through when pierced with a small knife or toothpick. If it is not ready, continue roasting and checking it every 10 minutes. You can let the cloves cook longer and get darker brown for a more caramelized flavor. Let cool and then squeeze the roasted garlic out of the skin into a small bowl and mash with a fork.

4. Preheat the oven to broil.

5. Toast the bread until just light brown.

6. Spread the roasted garlic on the lightly toasted bread.

7. Place on a baking sheet and broil on the highest rack for 1 minute or until the garlic and the bread are a little browned.

8. Remove from the oven, slice to desired size, and add salt (optional), pepper, and other seasonings to taste. Serve immediately.

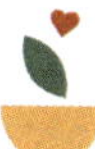

SAUTÉED GREENS

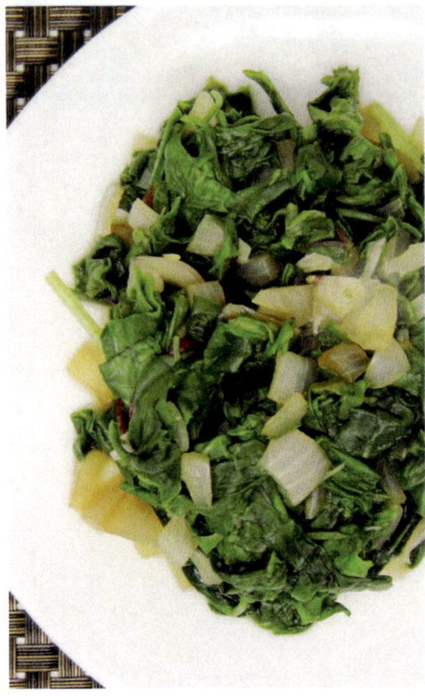

According to Dr. Caldwell Esselstyn, eating a handful of cooked, dark leafy greens once or twice a day is one of the most important things you can do for your health. I like to have a big bag of organic baby greens in my refrigerator all the time and shallots or onions on hand to sauté with them. I put a few spoonfuls of these cooked greens on baked beans, black beans, in bowls, in soups, and just on the side of my plate as often as possible (yes, even for breakfast). When I sauté the greens with shallots, I eat them just as they are, but you can sprinkle them with balsamic vinegar, WFPB hot sauce, or other flavorful sauces as well.

servings

2

4 cups finely chopped baby power greens or other dark, leafy greens of your choice

¼–⅓ cup diced shallot or onion

Salt and pepper to taste (eventually omit salt)

1. In a medium frying pan, water sauté the shallots or onions until soft. Then add the greens and sauté until wilted but still bright green. Serve right away.

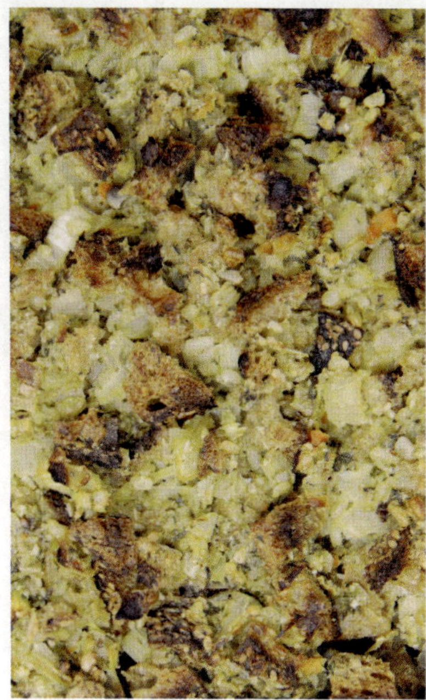

STUFFING

This aromatic sage, onion, and thyme stuffing is a great addition to a WFPB Thanksgiving dinner or just served with Mashed Potatoes (p 71), Gravy (p 94), and Sautéed Greens (p 76). You may want to dry out the bread cubes in the oven the day before to make things go more quickly on the day you make the stuffing. I like to put together all of the stuffing and let it sit overnight in the refrigerator, so the flavors blend before I bake it the next day.

1 large onion, diced (about 1 ½ cups)

3 celery stalks, diced

6 cups WFPB bread, chopped into cubes (about 8 slices of *Ezekiel 4:9* brand bread)

1 tbsp chopped fresh sage or to taste

2 tbsp chopped fresh thyme or to taste

2 cups vegetable broth, preferably low salt

Salt and pepper to taste (eventually omit salt)

1. Preheat oven to 250°F.

2. Spread the bread cubes in a single layer on a large baking sheet. Bake for 30 minutes.

3. Meanwhile, in a large pan, water sauté the onions and celery until soft and set aside.

4. When the bread cubes have baked for 30 minutes, remove them from the oven and stir. If the cubes are not dry enough, bake for another 30 minutes. If they are almost dry, switch the oven off and leave them in for another 15 minutes.

5. After removing the bread cubes, preheat the oven to 350°F.

6. Stir all of the ingredients into the onions and celery in the large pan. Then pour into an 11" x 7" oval casserole dish.

7. Bake for 45 minutes to an hour or until the top is brown and crisp.

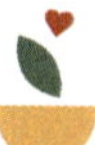

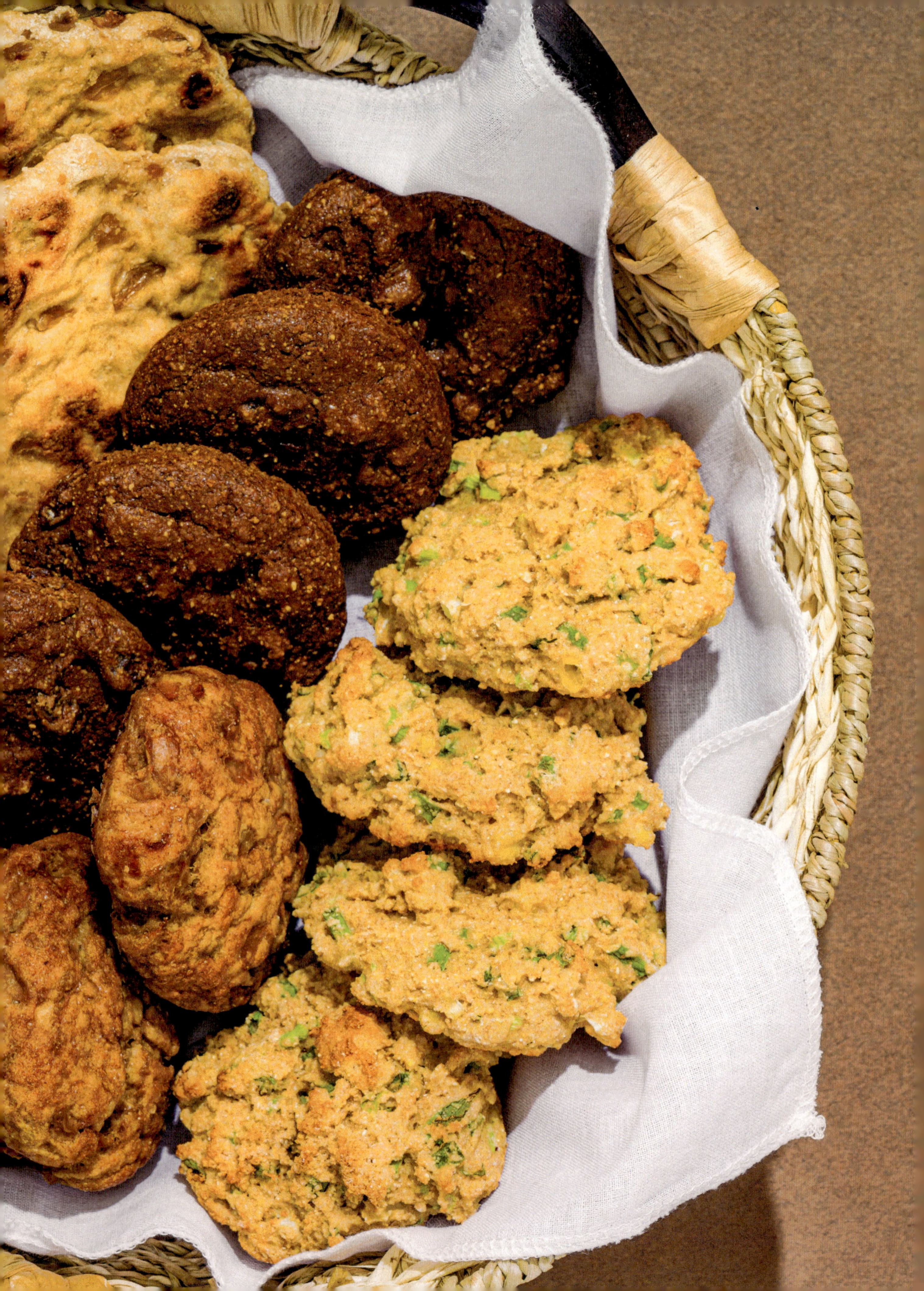

BREADS

There are some very good commercially sold WFPB breads, hamburger buns, and English muffins made by brands such as *Ezekiel 4:9*, *Engine 2*, and *Alvarado Street Bakery* among others. If you can't get these or you prefer homemade bread, the breads in this section are easy to make. The naan bread is great with gyros, falafel, and hummus. The caramelized onion burger buns are excellent for veggie burgers or sandwiches, and the pretzel rolls and cornbread biscuits are delicious with soups and salads. If you are not able to get whole spelt flour, you can replace it with whole wheat flour. I have recently started using sprouted whole wheat and whole spelt flour to enhance the nutritional value of the breads.

Using a bread machine to make the doughs for these breads is easiest; however, if you do not own a bread machine, follow these instructions to make any of the yeast breads:

1. Mix the non-dairy milk with the apple cider vinegar in a small bowl and let stand for 5 minutes.
2. In a large bowl, add the warm water to the yeast, stir, and let it rest for 5 minutes.
3. Add 1½ cups of the flour and the remaining ingredients (except caramelized onions) and mix on medium speed for 3 minutes.
4. Stir in another 1 cup of flour until the dough pulls away cleanly from the sides of the bowl.
5. On a floured surface, knead in the remaining ½ cup flour until the dough is smooth and elastic, about 10 minutes.
6. Place dough in a bowl, cover with a thin, cotton dishtowel and let rise in a warm place until doubled in bulk, about 30–45 minutes.
7. Punch down and follow instructions in the recipe for shaping and baking the bread.

BOSTON BROWN BREAD

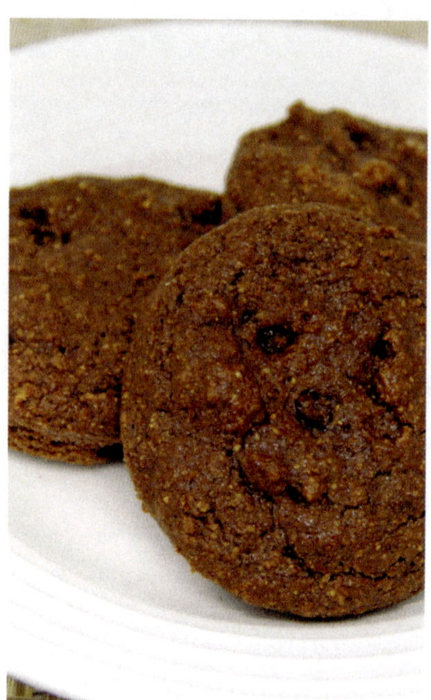

You can make this in a small Dutch oven or casserole dish with a cover (2 quart) or in a pudding mold. Whatever you use should fit into a large cooking pot because rather than being baked, this bread is steamed like what the British would call a pudding. This batter also makes excellent muffins or, if you prefer a chewier texture, muffin tops. Try topping with date-sweetened Cream Cheese (p 112) for a yummy snack or serve with Boston Baked Beans (p 41) and a side of Sautéed Greens (p 76).

1 cup unsweetened soy or other non-dairy milk

1 tbsp apple cider vinegar

½ cup rye flour

½ cup whole wheat flour

½ cup cornmeal

1 tsp baking soda

¾ tsp *salt* (gradually reduce)

⅓ cup *molasses*

½ cup raisins

servings

10–12

equipment

Parchment paper, muffin tin (optional), pudding mold (optional)

for one large loaf

1. Preheat oven to 325°F and bring a kettle of water to a boil.

2. In a small bowl, mix the non-dairy milk and apple cider vinegar and let stand for 5 minutes.

3. Combine the flours, cornmeal, baking soda, and salt in a bowl and whisk to mix.

4. Pour in the non-dairy milk mixture, molasses, and raisins and stir together.

5. Place parchment paper inside the Dutch oven or other baking dish. Pour the batter in and put the cover on.

6. Place the covered container into a deep pot and fill the pot with boiling water halfway up the side of the container. Do not put a lid on the large pot with the water. Place the pot with the container in it in the oven and bake for 2 hours. Occasionally check the water level in the pot and add more if needed.

7. Remove from the oven and stick a small knife or skewer down the center of the bread. If the bread is done, the knife will come out clean. If not, bake it a little longer.

8. Remove the container top and let the bread cool for about an hour before serving.

for muffins or muffin tops

1. Preheat oven to 350°F and bring a kettle of water to a boil.

2. In a small bowl, mix the non-dairy milk and apple cider vinegar and let stand for 5 minutes.

3. Combine the flours, cornmeal, baking soda, and salt in a bowl and whisk to mix.

4. Pour in the non-dairy milk mixture, molasses, and raisins and stir together.

5. Pour the batter into the nonstick muffin or muffin top tin. Use cupcake liners if you are worried about the muffins sticking to the tin.

6. Place the muffin tin in the middle of the oven with a wide bowl or pan full of boiling water on the shelf below and bake for 30 minutes or until a knife comes out clean.

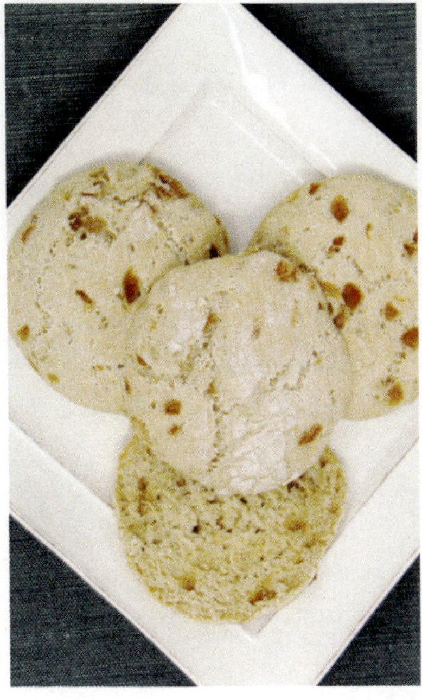

CARAMELIZED ONION BURGER BUNS

These are great with Veggie Burgers (p 62) and for other types of sandwiches. You can also leave out the caramelized onions for a more traditional burger bun.

Note that the Caramelized Onions (p 118) take 30–40 minutes to cook. I make a big batch of caramelized onions and freeze them in ½-cup servings to have them on hand for baking.

servings

10–12 buns

equipment

Parchment paper, bread machine (optional)

½ cup unsweetened soy or other non-dairy milk

1 tbsp apple cider vinegar

1¾ cups whole wheat pastry flour

1 ½ cups whole spelt flour (can be replaced with whole wheat flour)

2 ½ tsp active dry yeast

1 cup warm water

½ tsp *maple syrup*

½ tsp. *salt*

½ cup Caramelized Onions (p 118) (made from about 2 ½ cups diced onions)

1. In a small bowl, combine non-dairy milk and apple cider vinegar and let stand 5 minutes.

2. Add all ingredients except the onions to the bread machine and select the dough setting. If you do not have a bread machine, follow the instructions at the beginning of this section (p 79), noting when to add the onions in step 3 below.

3. If using a bread machine, add the caramelized onions directly to the dough in the bread machine after the first round of mixing or knead the onions into the dough on a floured board once it has completed its second rise and has been removed from the bread machine. If you are making the bread by hand, knead onions into the dough in the final punching down and shaping stage.

4. On a floured board, lightly knead the dough.

5. Divide the dough into 10–12 pieces, depending on how big you want the rolls to be. Roll them into balls, flatten them slightly and place on a piece of parchment paper on a baking sheet.

6. Cover with a thin, cotton dishtowel and let rise. For extra moist and fluffy dough, set the oven to 190°F for two minutes and turn it off. Then boil some water in a kettle and pour it into a shallow bowl or oven-proof baking dish. Place the covered buns on the top shelf of the oven and place the bowl of water beneath it. Close the oven door and let the dough rise for about half an hour or until the rolls have doubled in size.

7. When the rolls have risen, remove them from the oven and preheat the oven to 425°F. Bake for 12 minutes or until the bottoms are golden.

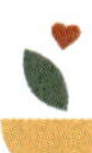

CARAMELIZED ONION NAAN BREAD

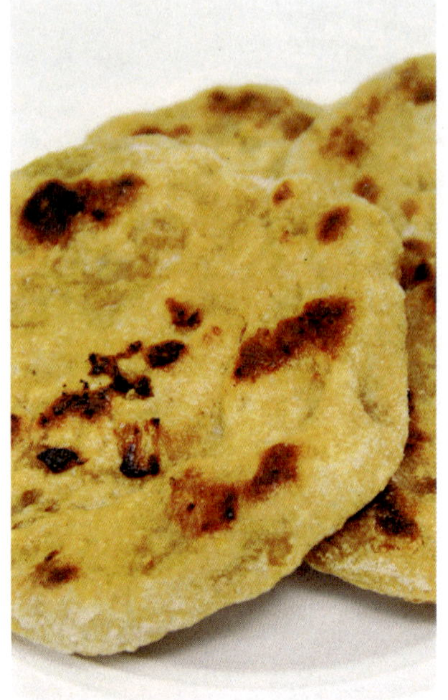

I can't get enough of these tasty flatbreads! I always have them in the freezer.

I dip them in Vegetable Curry (p 49), Dal (p 43), Hummus (p 96), and Tzatziki (p 105). The Caramelized Onions (p 118) give the bread a unique flavor that complements a variety of dishes. These are also delicious with Falafel (p 55) and Veggie Burgers (p 62). Try adding your favorite herbs and/or garlic for a change.

Note that the caramelized onions take 30–40 minutes to cook. I make a big batch of caramelized onions and freeze them in ½–cup servings to have them on hand for baking.

½ cup unsweetened soy or other non-dairy milk

1 tbsp apple cider vinegar

1¾ cups whole wheat pastry flour

1½ cups whole spelt flour (can be replaced with whole wheat flour)

1 tbsp malted barley flour (optional for a chewier texture)

2½ tsp active dry yeast

1 cup warm water

½ tsp *maple syrup*

¾ tsp *salt*

½ cup Caramelized Onions (p 118) (made from about 2 ½ cups diced onions)

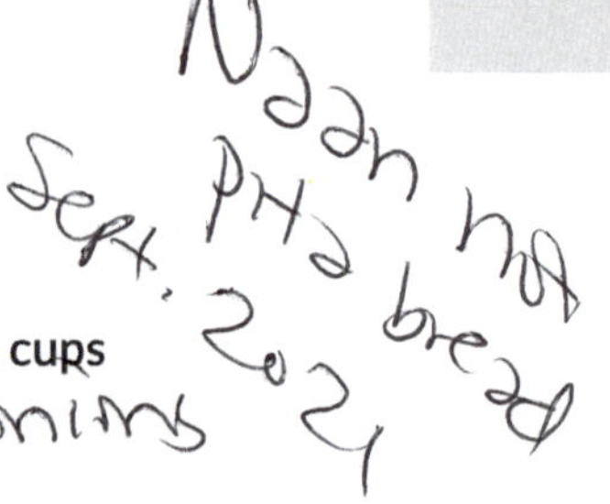

servings

24 small naan breads

equipment

Bread machine (optional), nonstick griddle

1. Combine non-dairy milk and apple cider vinegar in a small bowl and let stand 5 minutes.

2. Add all ingredients except the onions to the bread machine and select the dough setting. If you do not have a bread machine, follow the instructions at the beginning of this section (p 79).

3. If using a bread machine, add the caramelized onions directly to the dough in the bread machine after the first round of mixing or knead the onions into the dough on a floured board once it has completed its second rise and has been removed from the bread machine. If you are making the bread by hand, knead onions into the dough in the final punching down and shaping stage.

4. Preheat a nonstick griddle to 400°F.

5. On a floured board, lightly knead the dough.

6. Flatten golf ball-sized pieces of dough between two pieces of parchment paper, peel the dough off and place on the hot griddle, or flatten them directly onto the hot griddle. Let them cook about 4 minutes on each side or until they have some dark brown blisters on them.

Note: If you would prefer to make crispy onion naan bread crackers, cut the cooked naan bread rounds into 6 or 8 triangles and place on a baking sheet in the oven at 250°F for half an hour or until crisp.

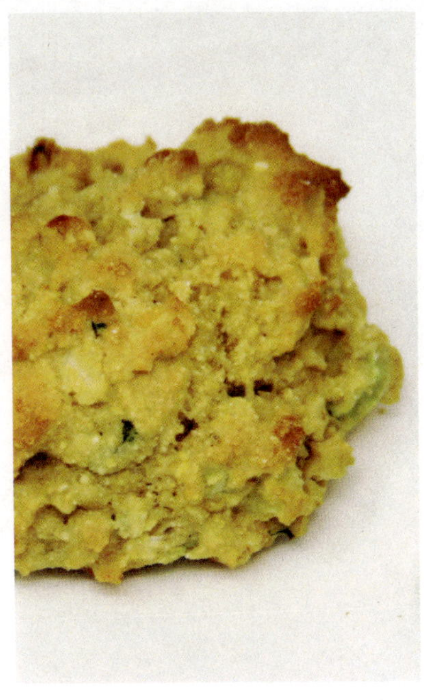

servings

12–15 biscuits

GREEN ONION & JALAPEÑO CORNBREAD BISCUITS

I absolutely love these biscuits crumbled over chili and other soups. The non-dairy milk and apple cider vinegar replace milk and eggs in traditional cornbread recipes. The corn, green onions, and jalapeño boost the nutritional value and add a nice southwestern flavor. Make a double batch and freeze them.

1 cup unsweetened soy or other non-dairy milk

1 tbsp apple cider vinegar

¾ cup cornmeal

1 tbsp soy or garbanzo bean miso (optional for flavor)

1 cup whole wheat pastry flour

½ cup almond flour

1 tbsp baking powder

¼ tsp baking soda

1 tsp *salt* (gradually reduce)

½ cup sliced green onions

½ cup thawed frozen corn or drained canned corn

2 tbsp minced jalapeño pepper (or to taste)

1. Preheat the oven to 450°F and line a baking sheet with parchment paper.

2. In a medium bowl, combine the non-dairy milk and the apple cider vinegar and let stand for 5 minutes.

3. Add the cornmeal and miso to the milk mixture and let stand for 15 minutes. Blend in the miso (with a fork or an immersion blender), so it does not stay in a clump.

4. In a large bowl, whisk together the flours, baking powder, baking soda, and salt. Add the green onions, corn, and jalapeño and mix.

5. Add the non-dairy milk mixture and stir until combined.

6. Drop ½-cup dollops onto the parchment paper on the baking sheet and bake for 12–14 minutes or until biscuits are golden brown on the bottom.

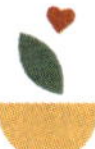

PIZZA DOUGH

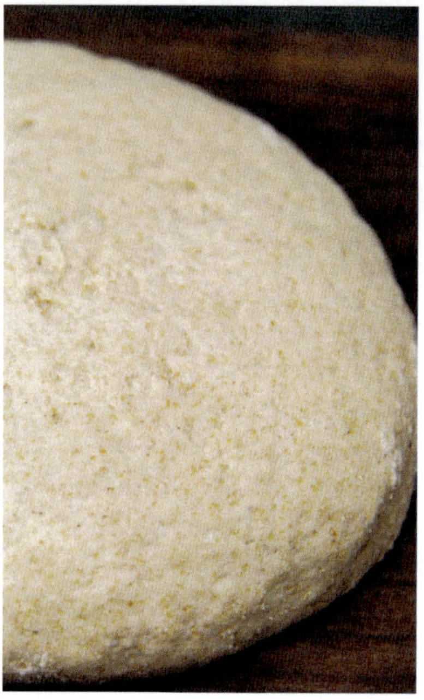

This double batch of dough is great for making two large pizzas with different toppings. If you only need to make one pizza, freeze or refrigerate the remaining dough until you need it. Refrigerate the dough if you will use it within 2–3 days.

½ cup unsweetened soy or other non-dairy milk

1 tbsp apple cider vinegar

1¾ cups whole wheat pastry flour

1½ cups whole spelt flour (can be replaced with whole wheat flour)

1 tbsp malted barley flour (optional, for texture)

2½ tsp active dry yeast

1 cup warm water

½ tsp *maple syrup*

¾ tsp *salt*

servings

2 pizza bases

equipment

Bread machine (optional), rolling pin

1. In a small bowl, combine the non-dairy milk and apple cider vinegar and let stand 5 minutes.

2. Add all ingredients to the bread machine and select the dough setting. If you do not have a bread machine, follow the instructions at the beginning of this section (p 79).

3. When ready, place the dough on a piece of parchment paper and flatten with a rolling pin into a thin, round circle (14"–16" in diameter).

4. Follow instructions in the Pizza recipes (pp 54, 59) to make WFPB pizza.

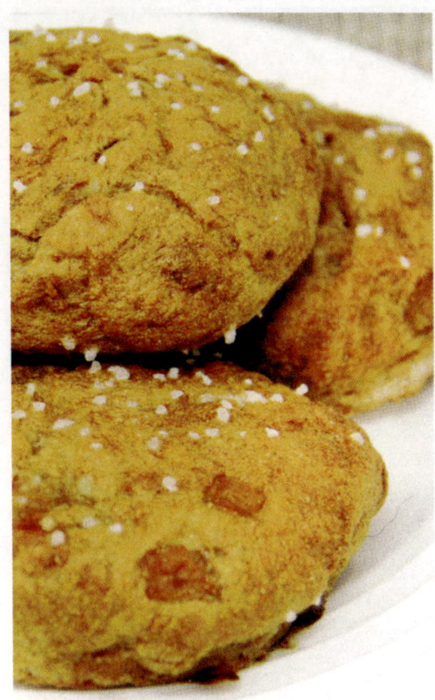

PRETZEL ROLLS

These are wonderful with Veggie Burgers (p 62), for savory sandwiches, or with soups. I like to add Caramelized Onions (p 118) to them for a nice sweet/savory combination. You can also make pretzel breadsticks and eat them with mustard.

Note that the caramelized onions take 30–40 minutes to cook. I make a big batch of caramelized onions and freeze them in ½-cup servings to have them on hand for baking.

½ cup unsweetened soy or other non-dairy milk

1 tbsp apple cider vinegar

1¾ cups whole wheat pastry flour

1½ cups whole spelt flour (can be replaced with whole wheat flour)

1 tbsp malted barley flour (optional for a chewier texture)

2½ tsp active dry yeast

1 cup warm water

½ tsp *maple syrup*

½ tsp *salt*

½ cup Caramelized Onions (p 118, optional, made from about 2½ cups diced onions)

5 cups water

2 tbsp baking soda

Coarse *salt* (gradually reduce or omit)

servings

12–16 rolls, depending on size

equipment

Bread machine (optioanl)

1. In a small bowl, combine non-dairy milk and apple cider vinegar and let stand 5 minutes.

2. Add all ingredients except the onions (if using) to the bread machine and select the dough setting. If you do not have a bread machine, follow instructions at the beginning of this section (p 79).

3. If using a bread machine, add the caramelized onions, if using, directly to the dough in the bread machine after the first round of mixing or knead the onions into the dough on a floured board once it has completed its second rise and has been removed from the bread machine; if you are making the bread by hand, knead onions into the dough in the final punching down and shaping stage.

4. Divide the dough into 12–16 pieces, depending on how big you want the rolls to be. Roll them into balls, flatten them slightly and place on a piece of parchment paper on a baking sheet.

5. Cover with a thin, cotton dishtowel and let rise. For extra moist and fluffy dough, set the oven to 190°F for two minutes and turn it off. Then boil some water in a kettle and pour it in a shallow bowl or cooking dish. Place the covered rolls on the top shelf of the oven and place the bowl of water beneath it. Close the oven door and let the dough rise for around half an hour or until doubled in size.

6. Meanwhile, in a large frying pan, bring the water and the baking soda to a boil.

7. When the rolls have risen, remove them from the oven, if you had them in the oven to rise, and preheat the oven to 425°F. Carefully place each roll upside down in the boiling baking soda water and leave it in for about 30 seconds. Lift out with a slotted spatula and drain as much water off as possible. Then place them back right side up on the parchment paper on the baking sheet.

8. Sprinkle the rolls lightly with coarse salt. Bake for 12 minutes or until golden on the bottom. You can cook them longer if you prefer a chewier, darker pretzel roll.

SAVORY CORNBREAD

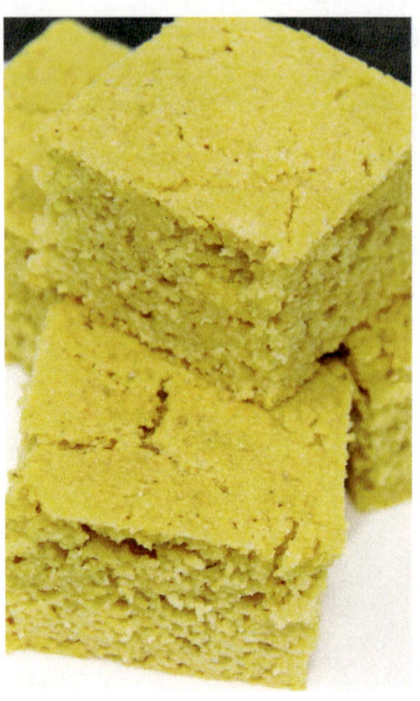

This moist and savory cornbread is wonderful with Black Bean and Corn Chili (p 40). The masa harina gives it a hint of tamale flavor and the whipped aquafaba creates a light texture.

1 cup unsweetened soy or other non-dairy milk

1 tbsp apple cider vinegar

¾ cup cornmeal

¾ cup masa harina

¼ cup whole wheat pastry flour

2 tsp baking powder

¼ tsp baking soda

½ tsp *salt* (gradually reduce)

⅓ cup water

½ cup aquafaba

servings

6–8

1. Preheat oven to 350°F.

2. In a medium bowl, add non-dairy milk and apple cider vinegar and let stand 5 minutes.

3. Add the cornmeal to the non-dairy milk mixture, stir with a fork, and let stand 10 minutes.

4. In a large bowl, combine the masa harina, whole wheat pastry flour, baking powder, baking soda, and salt.

5. In a medium bowl, whip the aquafaba until it forms stiff peaks.

6. Add the non-dairy milk mixture and water to the dry ingredients and stir until just mixed.

7. Fold the aquafaba into the batter.

8. Pour into a small square or round nonstick baking dish (about 8") and bake for 30 minutes.

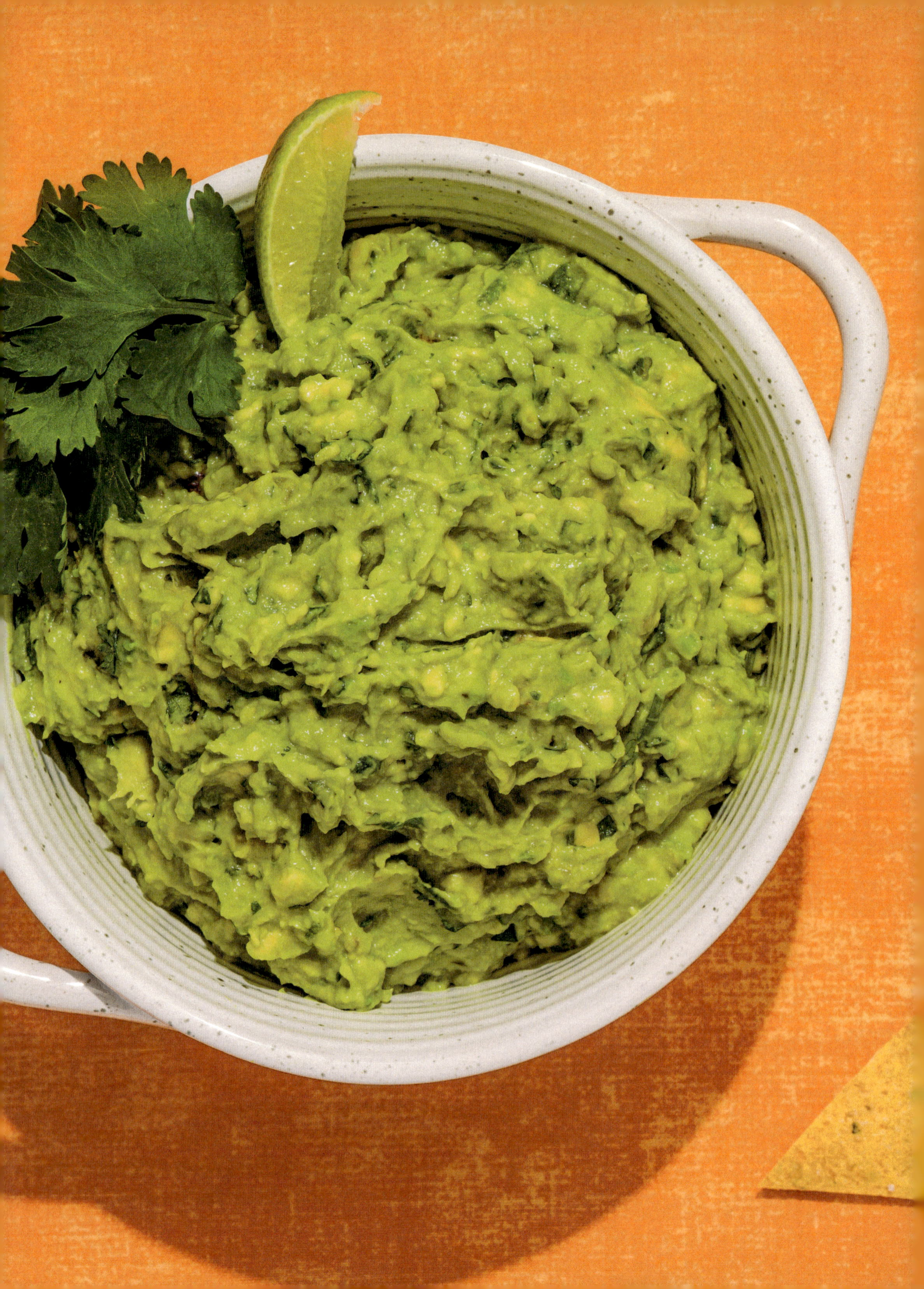

DIPS, SAUCES, AND SALAD DRESSINGS

Many commercial dips, sauces, and salad dressings are loaded with oils, thickeners, and even saturated fats. Enjoy these healthy dips with raw veggies, caramelized onion naan bread, or a WFPB cracker option like *Mary's Gone Crackers*. And the sauces are great for spicing up bowls and topping veggie stir fries and southwestern dishes. The best part is how quick and easy these recipes are to make!

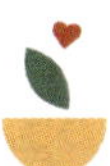

APPLE SAUCE

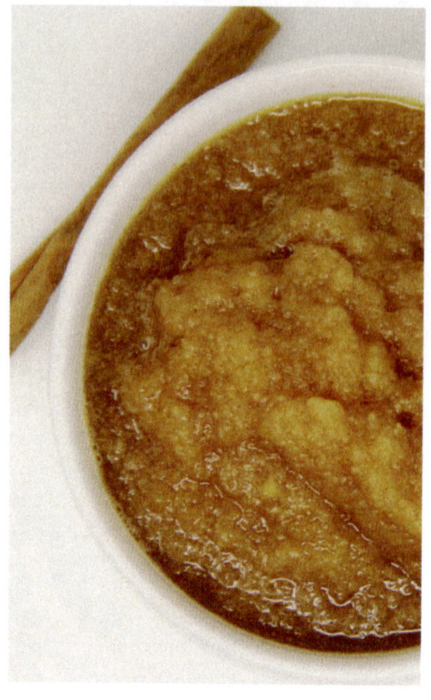

No, you don't have to cook apple sauce: just blend it! This is a really quick way to make a tasty side dish or topping for Potato Pancakes (p 72) or Oatmeal (p 132). The apple cider vinegar and cinnamon have heaps of health benefits. Use your favorite kind of apple as long as it is not too tart—I like Fuji apples.

4 medium apples, peeled, cored, and quartered

1 tbsp apple cider vinegar

1 tsp cinnamon (optional)

2 tbsp–¼ cup water (as needed for consistency)

servings

About 3 cups

equipment

Blender

1. Place all ingredients in a blender and blend 2–3 minutes or until smooth. Add water by the tablespoonful, as needed, for desired consistency. Store in a sealed container in the refrigerator.

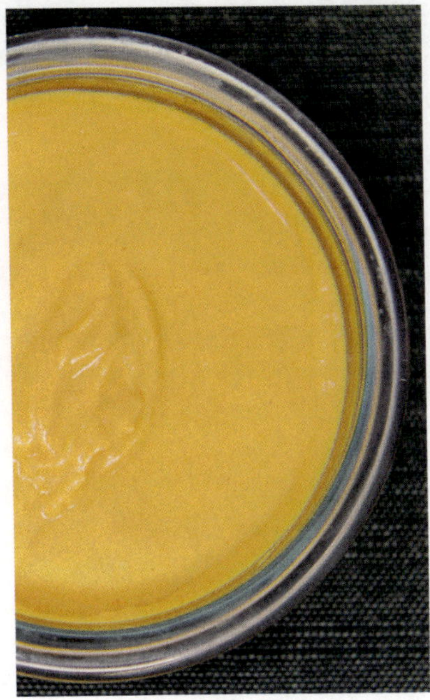

CHIPOTLE CREAM

This creamy, spicy sauce is delicious on Nachos (p 58) and can be used as a dip for raw veggies and Homemade Tortilla Chips (p 70).

½ cup Soaked Cashews (p 121)

¾ cup Salsa (p 101)

¼ tsp chili powder

¼ tsp *salt* (eventually omit)

1. Blend all ingredients in a bullet-style blender on high for 2–3 minutes or until smooth. Serve warm for nachos and chips and cold for fresh veggies.

servings

About 1 cup

equipment

Bullet-style blender

CRANBERRY RELISH

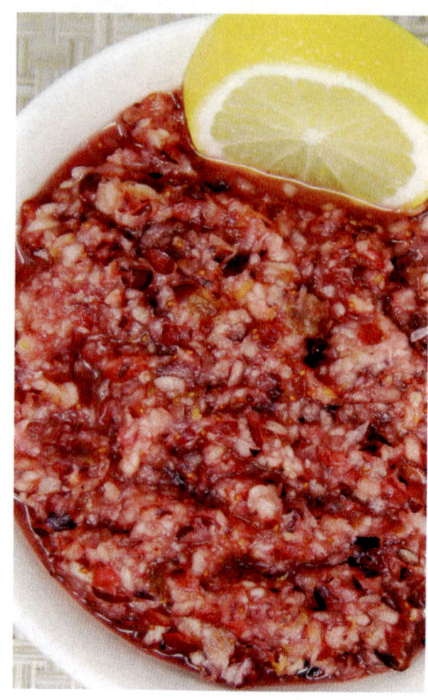

This fresh cranberry relish goes well with Mashed Potatoes (p 71), Stuffing (p 77), and Gravy (p 94). It is always on our holiday dinner table.

8 oz fresh cranberries

1 large, ripe orange (including zest)

1 small Fuji apple, peeled and cut into chunks

½ cup pitted, chopped medjool dates (add more for a sweeter relish)

servings

About 4 cups

1. Zest the orange, then discard the peel and cut it into chunks.

2. Add all ingredients to a food processor and pulse to desired texture. Store in a sealed glass container in the refrigerator.

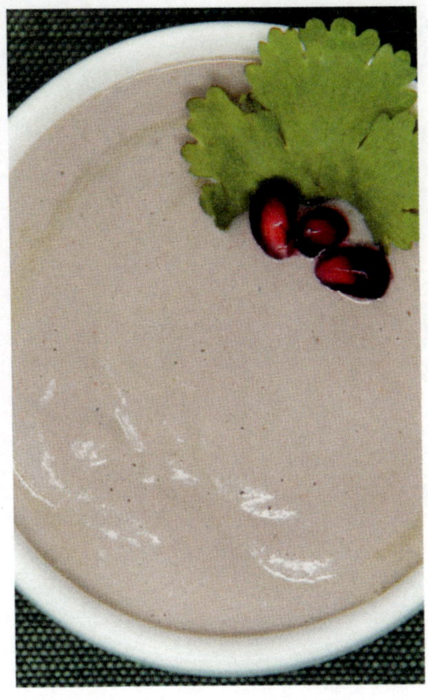

FRUITY CILANTRO SALAD DRESSING

This fruity, creamy dressing really helped me transition away from oily salad dressings. It is full of antioxidants from the strawberries, pomegranate seeds, and cilantro. It lasts 2–3 days in a sealed container in the refrigerator.

½ cup Sour Cream (p 102)

⅓ cup coarsely chopped cilantro leaves and stems

4–5 strawberries, hulled

¼–½ of a ripe pear

¼ cup pomegranate seeds

1. Blend all ingredients in a bullet-style blender for 1–2 minutes or until smooth.

servings

About 1 cup

equipment

Bullet-style blender

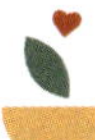

GRAVY

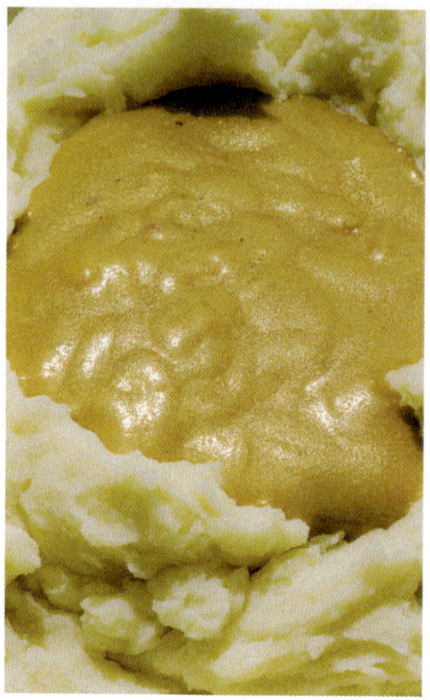

This gravy is a family favorite with Mashed Potatoes (p 71), Stuffing (p 77) and peas. Make the mushroom gravy for an even heartier meal.

Plain Gravy

2 cups water

½ cup Soaked Cashews (p 121)

2 tbsp *Bragg's Liquid Aminos* (use less if you are trying to reduce salt)

2 tbsp *tapioca flour*

1 tsp onion powder

1 tsp nutritional yeast

Dash of white pepper

1 tsp chopped fresh thyme (optional for more flavor)

½ tsp chopped fresh sage (optional for more flavor)

1. Add all of the ingredients to a bullet-style blender and blend 1–2 minutes or until smooth.

2. Pour the liquid into a medium saucepan and cook on medium heat for 3–5 minutes, stirring constantly until the gravy thickens to the desired consistency.

Mushroom Gravy

1 cup sliced mushrooms

¼ cup diced shallot

1. Blend all of the ingredients for the plain gravy in a bullet-style blender and set aside.

2. In a medium saucepan, water sauté the shallots for 2 minutes, then add the mushrooms and sauté for another 2–3 minutes.

3. Add the plain gravy mixture to the mushrooms and shallots in the saucepan and cook over medium heat for 3–5 minutes, stirring constantly until the gravy thickens to the desired consistency.

servings

About 2 cups

equipment

Bullet-style blender

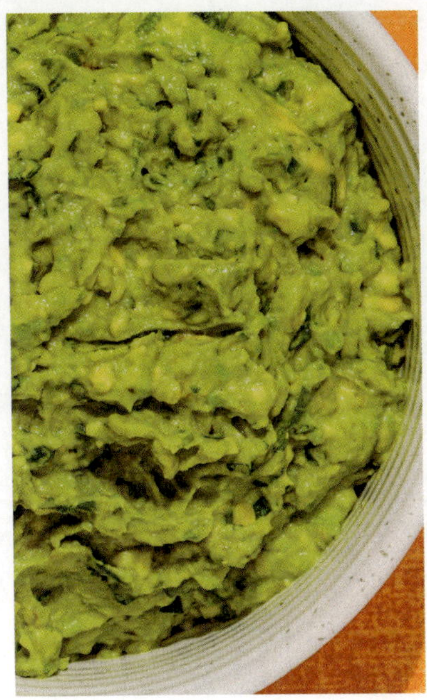

servings

6 servings

GUACAMOLE

This guacamole is great on Nachos (p 58), Bean and Cheese Quesadillas (p 53), Southwestern Bowls (p 34) and Nacho Salads (p 26). Try dipping Homemade Tortilla Chips (p 70) in it, too!

3 ripe avocados

¼–⅓ cup finely minced onion

1 tbsp finely minced fresh jalapeño pepper (or to taste)

¼ cup finely minced cilantro

2 tsp fresh squeezed lime juice (or to taste)

Salt and pepper to taste (eventually omit salt)

1. Peel avocados and remove pits.

2. In a medium bowl, mash the avocados to the desired consistency.

3. Add the remaining ingredients except for salt and pepper, and stir in with a fork.

4. Add salt (optional) and pepper to taste.

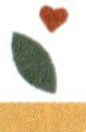

HUMMUS

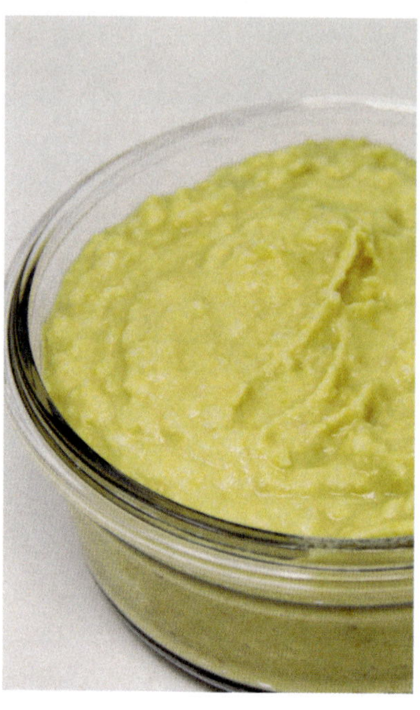

Hummus can be costly to buy, but it is easy and inexpensive to make. Try adding your favorite herbs and spices to the basic recipe. Use as a dip for vegetables, crackers, and Caramelized Onion Naan Bread (p 82), or as a spread for toast or sandwiches.

I find a food processor works better than a blender for hummus. Store in a sealed container in the refrigerator.

3 cups cooked Garbanzo Beans (p 119) or 2 cans (15 oz) garbanzo beans, ½ cup cooking liquid reserved

⅓ cup chopped sweet or yellow onion

¼ cup tahini

2 tbsp lemon juice

1 clove garlic

½ tsp *salt* (gradually reduce)

Roasted Garlic and/or Caramelized Onion variation

1 head of roasted garlic (omit raw garlic if you use this)

and/or

½ cup caramelized onions (omit raw onion if you use this)

servings

6

equipment

Food processor or blender

For Kalamata Olive variation

(note: this variation has the most salt)

10 whole kalamata olives

10 chopped kalamata olives

For Cilantro and Jalapeño variation

⅓ cup loosely packed fresh cilantro leaves and stems

1 small jalapeño pepper, seeded and chopped or to taste

For Roasted Garlic/Caramelized Onion and Cilantro/Jalapeño variations

1. Add all ingredients to a food processor or blender and start blending on low. Then gradually turn up the speed and blend until smooth.

For Kalamata Olive variation

1. Add all ingredients except the chopped olives to the food processor or blender and start blending on low. Then gradually turn up the speed and blend until smooth.

2. Stir in the chopped olives.

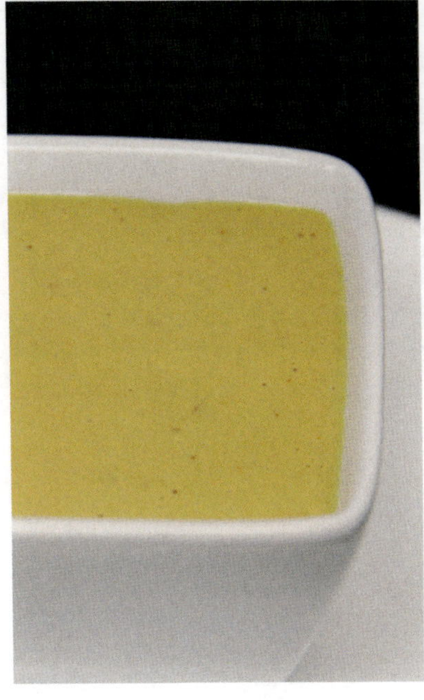

INDONESIAN PEANUT SAUCE

This high protein sauce is wonderful on tofu, tempeh, stir fries and bowls. The red pepper flakes give it a nice zing.

servings

About ¾ cup

equipment

Bullet-style blender

⅓ cup coarsely chopped yellow or sweet onion

2 medium cloves garlic

½ cup peanut butter without added oils or sugars or ¾ cup unsalted peanuts

¾ tsp fresh grated ginger

¼ tsp red pepper flakes or to taste

1 tbsp tamari, preferably low salt

¼ tsp *maple syrup*

2 tbsp fresh squeezed lime juice

⅓ cup boiling water

1. Blend all ingredients in a bullet-style blender. Add additional water by the tablespoonful, if needed, to achieve desired thickness.

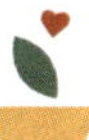

KOREAN STYLE HOT SAUCE

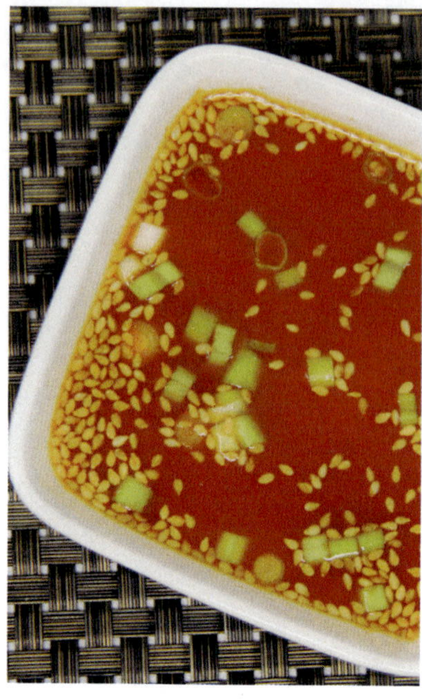

This is a great sauce for stir fries and bowls. It can also be used as a marinade for tofu or tempeh. Make a double batch and keep the extra in the refrigerator or freezer.

2 tbsp Korean chili paste (gochujang, make sure it has no MSG)

1 medium garlic clove, pressed

1 tbsp rice vinegar

1 tbsp soy sauce or tamari, preferably low salt

1 tbsp toasted sesame seeds

2 green onions, finely chopped

¼ tsp *maple syrup*

Boiling water

servings

½ cup

1. In a small bowl, stir together all ingredients with a fork, adding boiling water to achieve desired consistency.

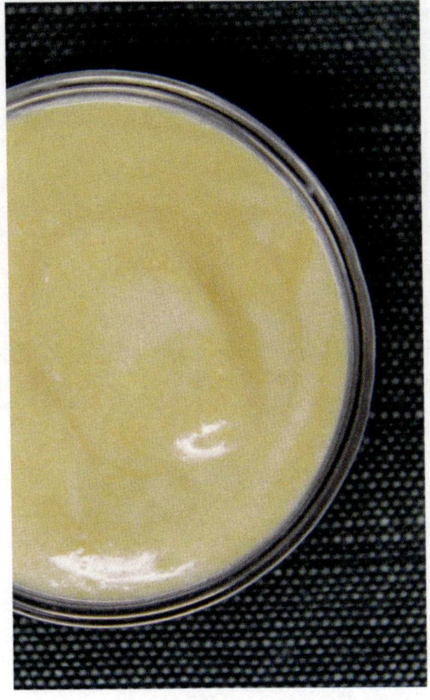

MISO DRESSING

This is a great dressing for Asian Bowls (p 32) or salads. Make a double batch and keep the extra in the refrigerator.

1 tbsp toasted black or white sesame seeds

2 tbsp miso, preferably low salt

2 tbsp rice vinegar

1 tbsp tamari, preferably low salt

½ tsp fresh grated ginger

½ cup water

¼ cup Soaked Cashews (p 121)

servings

About 1 cup

equipment

Bullet-style blender

1. If you don't have toasted sesame seeds, preheat the oven the 350°F. Place raw sesame seeds on a small baking tray and bake for 3 minutes or until lightly toasted.

2. Add all ingredients to a bullet-style blender and blend 1–2 minutes or until smooth. Add more water by the tablespoonful, if needed, to achieve desired consistency.

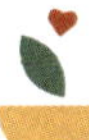

NACHO BEAN DIP

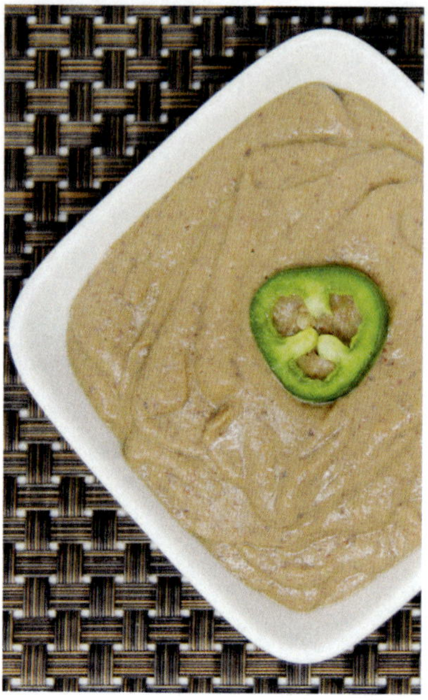

I love using Spicy Black Beans (p 122) for this and drizzling it on Nachos (p 58), Nacho Salad (p 26), and steamed plantains. It is also a great dip for parties. Serve along with Salsa (p 101), Guacamole (p 95), and Homemade Tortilla Chips (p 70).

1 can (15 oz) black beans, preferably low salt, or 1 ½ cups homemade (p 119, spicy optional), drained and rinsed (optional: reserve ¼ cup cooking liquid)

½ cup Nacho Cheese Sauce (p 111)

1–2 tbsp chopped jalapeño

¼ cup chopped sweet onion

¼ cup water or cooking liquid from beans

¼ tsp *salt* (eventually omit)

servings

About 1 ¾ cups

equipment

Bullet-style blender

1. Blend all ingredients in a bullet-style blender.

Note: If you don't have spicy black beans, you can add the following to a can of regular black beans: 1 tsp garlic powder, 1 tsp cumin, ½ tsp chili powder.

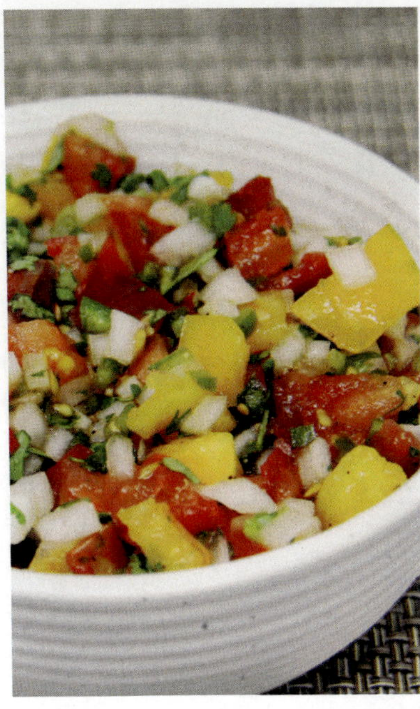

SALSA

This nutrient packed salsa is great for topping Nachos (p 58), Nacho Salad (p 26), and Southwestern Bowls (p 34). Try adding other ingredients like diced ripe mango or jicama for variety.

servings

6

3 ripe tomatoes, finely diced

1 medium onion, diced (about 1 cup)

2 jalapeños, seeded and diced (about ¼ cup or to taste)

½ cup chopped cilantro

2 tsp lime juice or to taste

Salt and pepper to taste (eventually omit salt)

1. Mix everything in a bowl. Store in a sealed container in the refrigerator.

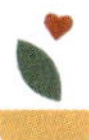

SOUR CREAM

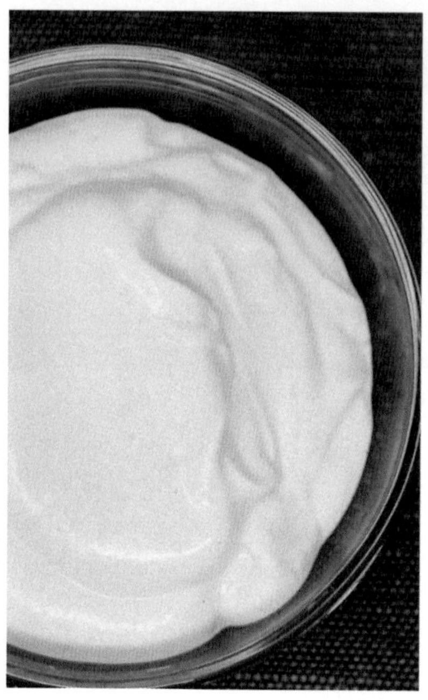

This is a key ingredient in Potato Salad (p 27) and a number of dips and sauces. It is also great for garnishing Nachos (p 58), soups, and even Potato Pancakes (p 72). Leftover sour cream can be kept in a sealed container in the refrigerator or freezer.

1 cup Soaked Cashews (p 121)

⅓ cup fresh lemon juice

¼ tsp salt (eventually omit)

1 tsp nutritional yeast

¼–⅓ cup water

servings

About 1 cup

equipment

Bullet-style blender

1. Add all ingredients to a bullet-style blender and blend on high for 2–3 minutes or until smooth and creamy. Add a few more cashews for a thicker, fluffier sour cream or more water for a thinner, crema-style cream.

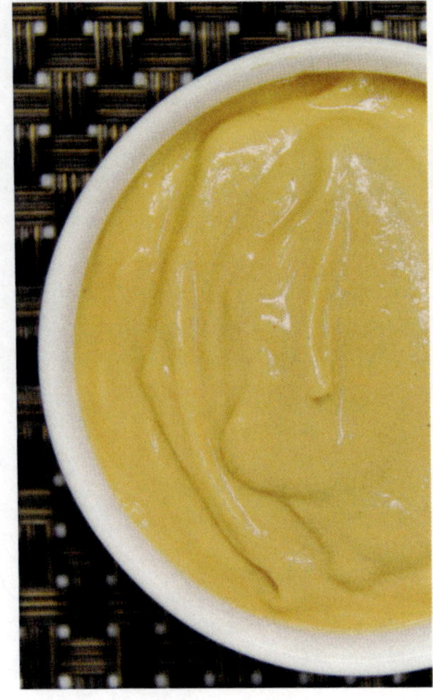

SPECIAL SAUCE FOR VEGGIE BURGERS

This sauce is a WFPB version of the types of sauces that come on fast food burgers. If you find yourself craving that type of food, slathering this sauce on a Veggie Burger (p 62) and eating it with Air Fried French Fries or Sweet Potato Fries (p 68) can be a healthy and enjoyable substitute. Don't forget to have a salad or greens with it as well! Store in a sealed container in the refrigerator or freezer.

1 large pitted, chopped medjool date

¼ cup boiling water

½ cup Soaked Cashews (p 121)

3 tbsp tomato paste, low salt if possible

1 tbsp mustard

1 tbsp white vinegar

¼ cup chopped sweet onion

Pinch of *salt* (eventually omit)

1. In a small bowl, add the boiling water to the chopped date, cover and let stand 5 minutes.

2. Add all ingredients to a bullet-style blender and blend 1–2 minutes or until smooth and creamy.

servings

About 1 cup

equipment

Bullet-style blender

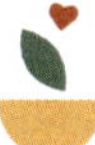

TAHINI DRESSING

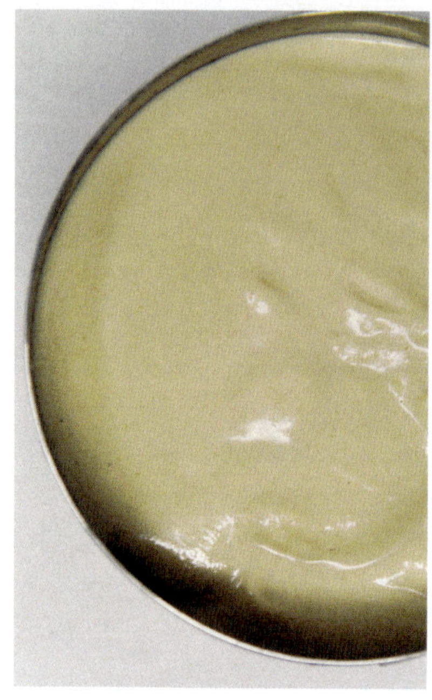

This is a great dressing for salads and Middle Eastern (p 33) or Asian Bowls (p 32). Make a double batch and keep it in sealed container in the refrigerator.

¼ cup tahini

1 small clove garlic

2 tbsp lemon juice

¼ cup Soaked Cashews (p 121)

1 tbsp tamari, preferably low salt

½ tsp *maple syrup*

¼–⅓ cup water

servings

½–¾ cup

equipment

Bullet-style blender

1. Add all ingredients to a bullet-style blender and blend for 1–2 minutes or until smooth. Add more water by the tablespoonful, if needed, to achieve desired consistency.

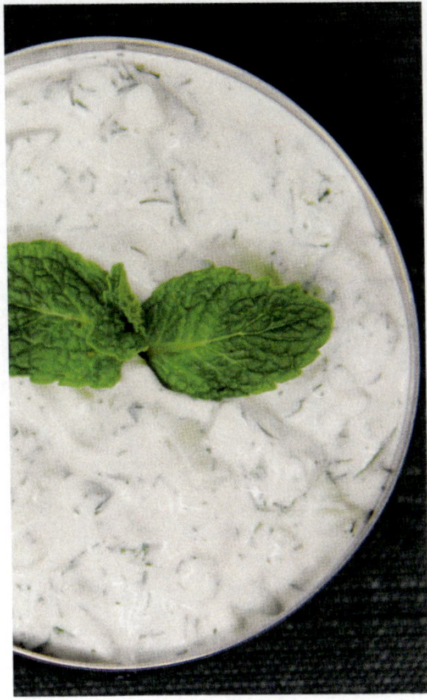

TZATZIKI

This sauce is delicious on Middle Eastern Bowls (p 33), Mushroom and Bell Pepper Gyros (p 60), and Falafel (p 55) and as a dip for Caramelized Onion Naan Bread (p 82) or vegetables. Store in a sealed container in the refrigerator.

servings

About 2 cups

equipment

Bullet-style blender

1 cup Soaked Cashews (p 121)

3 tbsp fresh lemon juice

¼–⅓ cup water (less water for thicker texture)

1 tsp nutritional yeast

Pinch of *salt*

2 small cucumbers, finely diced

2 tbsp minced fresh dill

2 tbsp minced fresh mint

2 tbsp minced fresh parsley

1. Blend the cashews, lemon juice, water, nutritional yeast, and salt in a bullet-style blender 2–3 minutes or until smooth.

2. Pour the cashew mixture in a medium bowl and stir in the cucumber, dill, mint, and parsley.

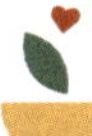

WORCESTERSHIRE SAUCE

This sauce adds flavor to a variety of dishes and is a nice marinade for mushrooms, tofu, and tempeh.

Note: traditional Worcestershire sauce contains anchovies and so is not WFPB. If you don't have time to make it yourself, there are brands at health food stores that do not have anchovies. Be careful not to get a sauce with MSG in it.

1 cup apple cider vinegar

⅓ cup dark *molasses*

¼ cup tamari

¼ cup water

3 tbsp lemon juice

1 tsp *salt* (gradually reduce)

1 ½ tsp dry mustard powder

1 tsp onion powder

¾ tsp ground ginger

½ tsp black pepper

¼ tsp garlic powder

¼ tsp cayenne pepper

⅛ tsp ground allspice

servings

About 2 cups

equipment

Bullet-style blender

1. Blend all of the ingredients in a bullet-style blender.

2. Pour the mixture into a medium saucepan and bring it to a boil, then immediately remove from the heat. Store in a sealed container in the refrigerator.

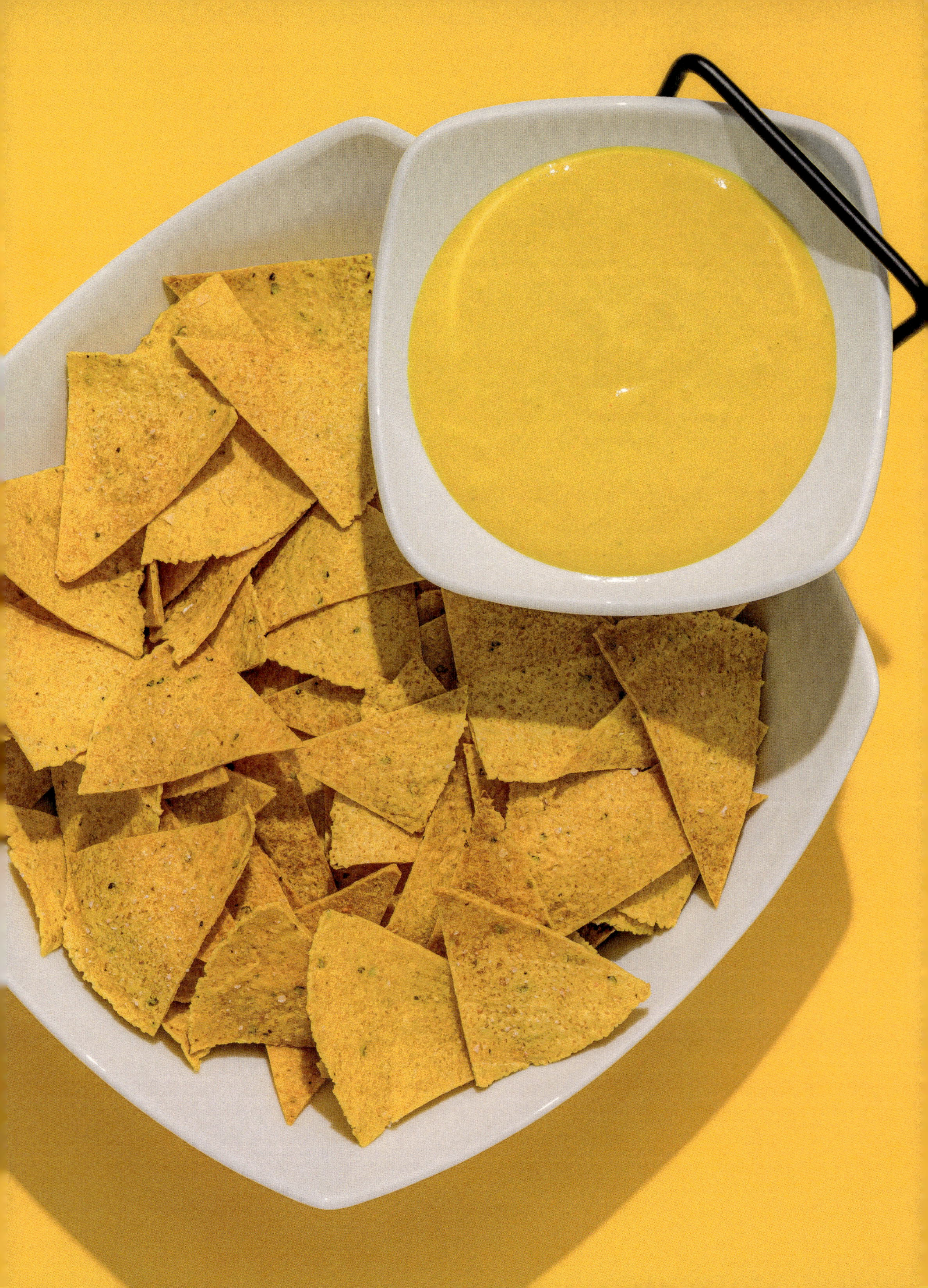

CHEESES

Many people I know who have switched to eating WFPB or vegan have said that cheese was the last thing to go. I too was sad to let go of my favorite Swiss cheese and Brie. But I have since discovered a nice variety of homemade WFPB cheeses that take the place of some of the cheeses that are vital components of some of our favorite foods, such as pizza, nachos, quesadillas, and more. In time, your taste buds adjust and you will find yourself enjoying these foods as much as you did the ones with dairy cheese, but without the consequences of eating all of the saturated fat.

Please note that many commercially sold vegan cheeses contain a lot of oil and would not be considered WFPB.

Almond Ricotta Cheese
110

Nacho Cheese Sauce
111

Cream Cheese
112

Fermented Cream Cheese
113

Mozzarella
114

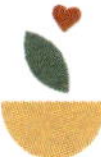

ALMOND RICOTTA CHEESE

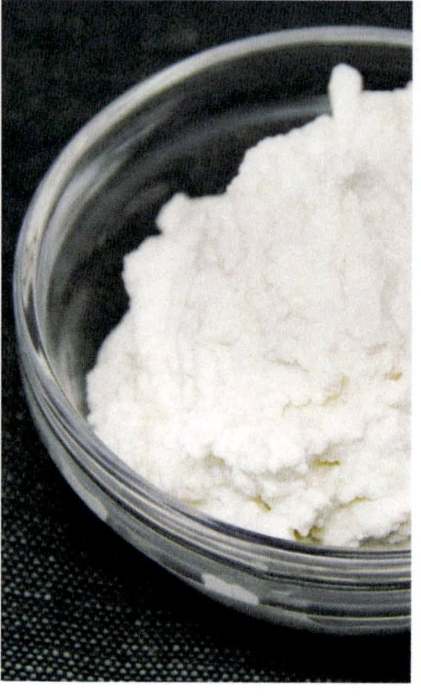

This cheese is delicious on the Butternut Squash and Caramelized Onion Pizza (p 54). I like to make a double batch and keep it in the freezer in 1-cup servings.

2 cups blanched almonds*, soaked overnight

1 cup water

Pinch of *salt* (optional, eventually omit)

1. Put everything in a bullet-style blender or food processor and blend until ricotta texture is achieved.

*If you can't find blanched almonds at the store, you can make them yourself from raw almonds with the skin on. Bring a pot of water to a boil on the stove and put 2 cups of almonds in the boiling water for 1 minute. Immediately drain and transfer the almonds into cold water, then gently squeeze the almonds to pop them out of their skins.

servings

About 1 ½ cups

equipment

Bullet-style blender or food processor

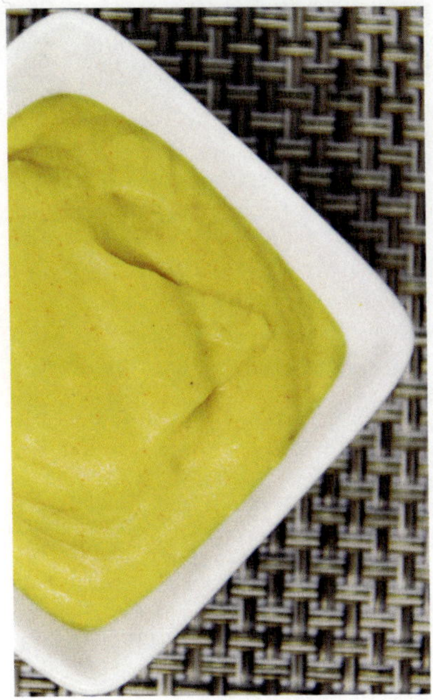

NACHO CHEESE SAUCE

This cheese sauce is great in Bean and Cheese Quesadillas (p 53) or drizzled warm over Nachos (p 58). Add minced jalapeños if you like it spicy.

½ cup Soaked Cashews (p 121)

2 tbsp *tapioca flour*

2 tsp lemon juice

1 tsp apple cider vinegar

1 ¼ cups water

2 tbsp nutritional yeast

1 tsp miso, preferably low salt

½ tsp paprika

½ tsp garlic powder

¼ tsp turmeric

⅛ tsp white pepper

1 tbsp diced jalapeño pepper (optional if you like it hot)

1. Blend the soaked cashews and all other ingredients in a bullet-style blender for 2 minutes or until smooth. You can add the jalapeños now (if using) if you want them blended in and cooked into the cheese.

2. Pour the mixture into a medium saucepan and cook over medium heat for 5 minutes or until the cheese sauce thickens, stirring constantly to prevent sticking. You can also add jalapeños now (if using) if you want larger, less cooked pieces in the cheese sauce.

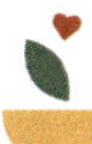

CREAM CHEESE

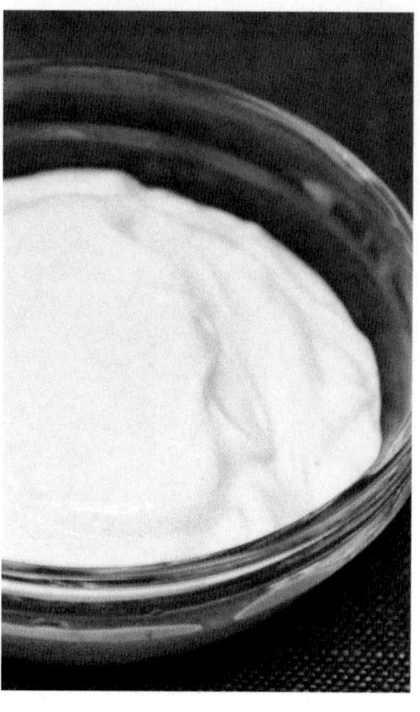

This cream cheese is nice on sprouted whole grain bagels or toast with veggies or fruit spread. Sweeten it with dates and spread it on Pumpkin Cranberry Bread (p 133) or toasted Boston Brown Bread (p 80), or add chives, olives, or jalapeños to make a zesty, savory version.

2 cups Soaked Cashews (p 121)

½ cup water

¼ cup fresh lemon juice

Pinch *salt* (eventually omit)

Sweet Cream Cheese

½ cup pitted, chopped, medjool dates, soaked in ½ cup boiling water (omit ½ cup water above)

Savory Cream Cheese

¼ cup finely minced chives

Or

¼ cup finely chopped green olives

Or

¼ cup finely chopped cilantro

2 tsp finely minced jalapeño

servings

About 1 ½ cups

equipment

Bullet-style blender

1. Blend cashews, water, lemon juice, and salt in a bullet-style blender until smooth. For a thicker consistency, add soaked cashews by the tablespoon and blend.

2. For a sweet version, add dates with the other ingredients.

3. For a savory version, omit dates and stir in any ingredients for the savory cream cheese after the cheese is blended.

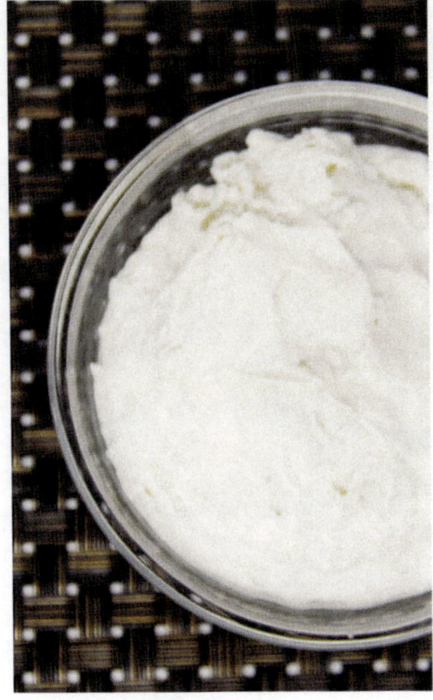

FERMENTED CREAM CHEESE

This has a slightly milder flavor than the Cream Cheese (p 112). Add herbs for a savory spread or dates for a sweet spread for Boston Brown Bread (p 80), Pumpkin Cranberry Bread (p 133), or Cinnamon Rolls (p 130).

servings

About 1 ½ cups

2 cups Soaked Cashews (p 121)

½ cup water

2 tbsp plain, non-dairy yogurt

Pinch *salt* (eventually omit)

1. Blend all ingredients until smooth.

2. Pour into a glass storage container with an airtight lid and let ferment for a day at room temperature. If it is not tangy enough, let it ferment for 1 more day.

3. Store in a sealed glass container in the refrigerator.

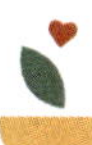

MOZZARELLA

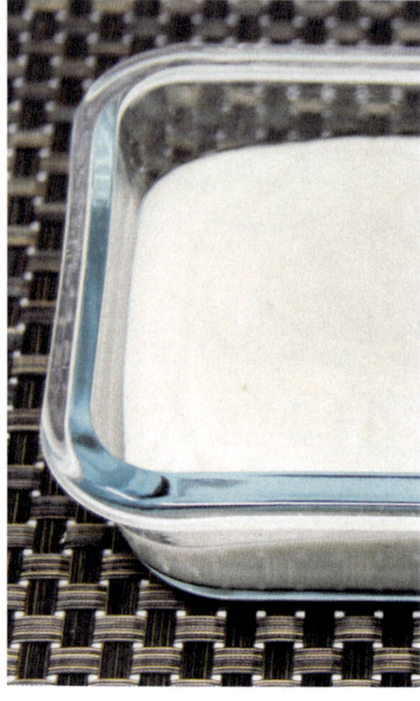

I like to make a large pot of this cheese and freeze it in small containers so I have it anytime I want to make Pizza (p 59) or Bean and Cheese Quesadillas (p 53).

Note: this cheese is too soft at room temperature to slice. It is best for melting on pizzas or quesadillas and is not suitable for cold dishes such as Caprese salad.

½ cup Soaked Cashews (p 121)

2 tbsp *tapioca flour*

1 tsp lemon juice

1 ¼ cup water

1 ½ tbsp nutritional yeast

¾ tsp *salt* (eventually omit)

½ tsp garlic powder

¼ tsp white pepper

About 1 ½ cups

Bullet-style blender or food processor

1. Blend all ingredients in a bullet-style blender for 2 minutes or until smooth.

2. Pour the cashew mixture into a saucepan. Cook over medium heat for 5 minutes or until the cheese thickens, stirring constantly to prevent sticking.

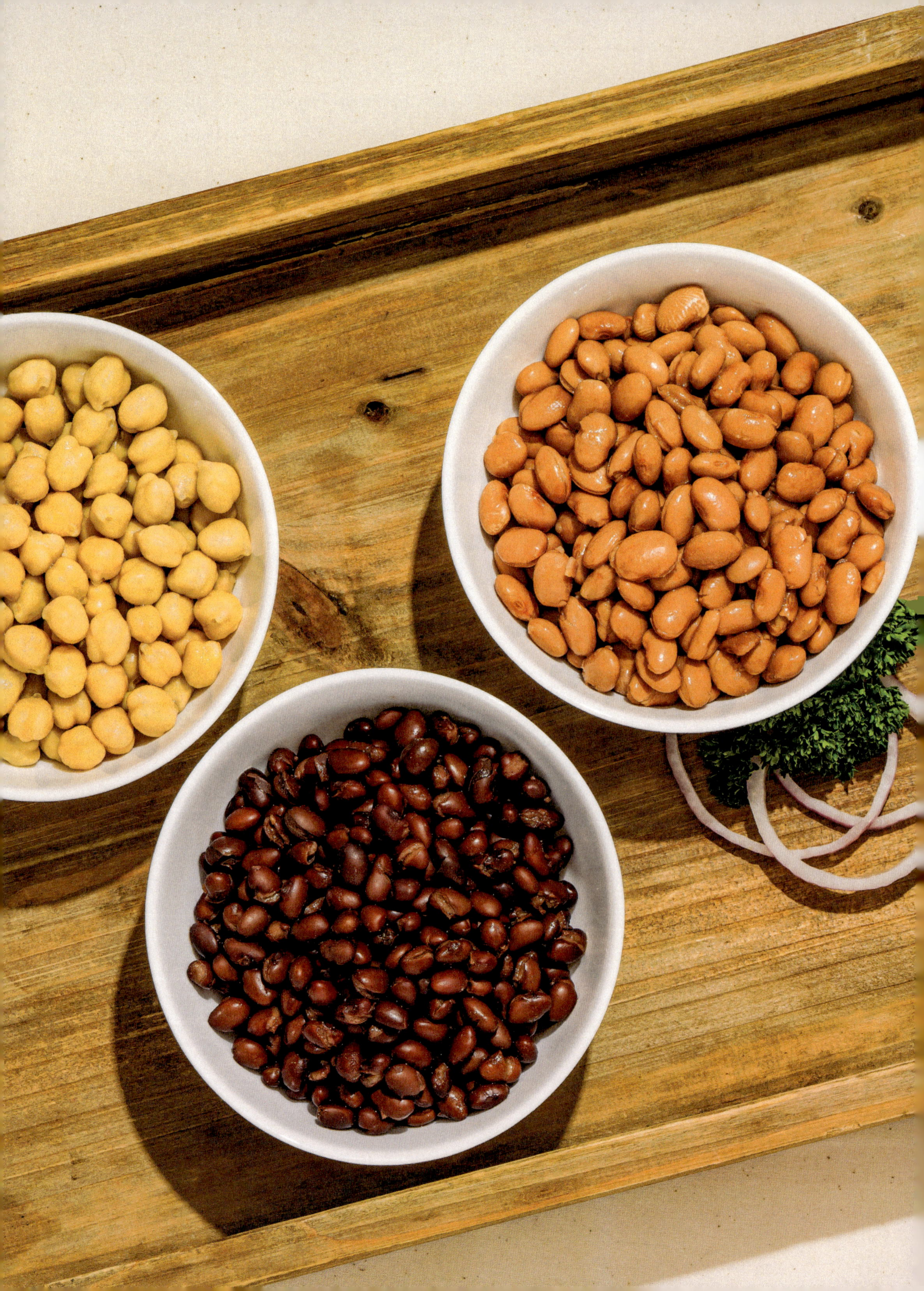

STAPLES

Staples are foods that are used in a lot of the recipes in this book and can be made inexpensively in bulk and stored in the refrigerator or freezer. Making these foods yourself ensures that you know exactly what is in them, and you can customize them to your taste. Making one or two of these a week will help you build up a convenient stock of your favorite foods and ingredients.

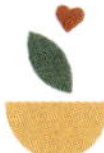

CARAMELIZED ONIONS

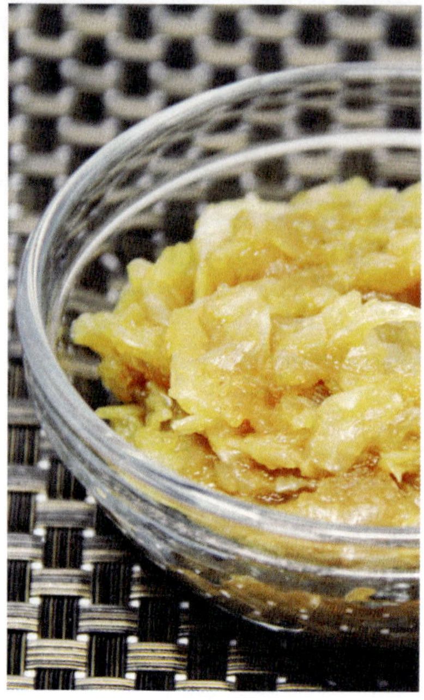

These are great on Pizza (p 59), in Caramelized Onion Naan Bread (p 82), Caramelized Onion Burger Buns (p 81), Pretzel Rolls (p 85), and Hummus (p 96). I use them so often that I caramelize four onions at a time and freeze them in ½-cup servings for easy use.

4 large onions, diced (about 6 cups)

Water

1. Over medium heat, water sauté the onions (without oil), adding small amounts of water each time they begin to get dry. Cook them 20–30 minutes. Towards the end, let them get a little brown so that when you add the water, it turns the entire mixture brown.

servings

About 2 cups

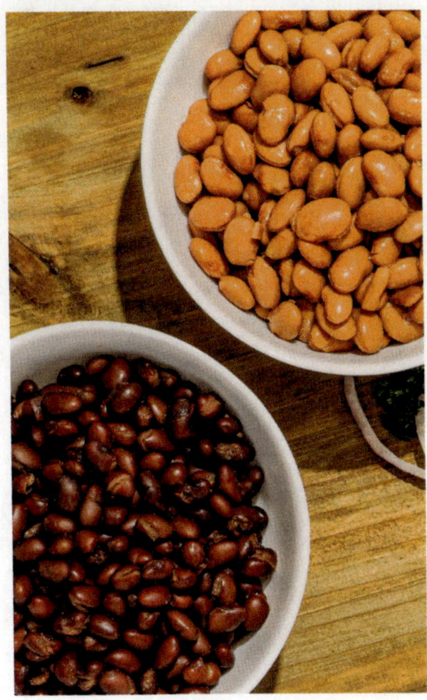

COOKED BEANS

Cooking beans at home can reduce the amount of food you are eating from cans—and it's really easy! This recipe can be used for any type of bean that you wish to use in soups, bowls, chilis, or on salads. Beans that I recommend keeping on hand are garbanzo, navy, cannellini, great northern, pinto, black, chili, and kidney beans. They are easy to make and will last a long time in the refrigerator or freezer. You can add your favorite herbs and spices as well: for example, I like adding Italian seasoning to the white beans and cumin to black beans.

servings

6 cups

equipment

Pressure cooker or Instant Pot

2 cups dried beans

Water

Your favorite herbs and spices (optional)

Pinch of baking soda (if your water is really hard, i.e., full of minerals)

1. Soak the beans in cold water overnight at room temperature, 8–12 hours. Soaking beans too long can cause the skins to toughen.

2. Rinse thoroughly in a strainer and place in a pot with water to an inch above the beans. Add herbs and spices if desired.

3. Bring to a boil, add the pinch of baking soda if your water is hard, and then reduce to a simmer, cooking the beans 1–2 hours or until just tender. Test them after 45 minutes and then every 10–15 minutes. The best way to test for doneness is to either cut or bite a bean in half: there should be no white left at the center. You can also cook the beans more quickly by using a pressure cooker or Instant Pot.

Note: be sure to save the water from your cooked garbanzo beans. This is aqua faba and is an ingredient in a number of recipes in this cookbook.

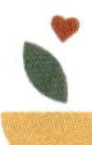

PIZZA SAUCE

This zesty sauce is great to make in large batches and freeze in pizza-sized servings. I always have plenty of this and frozen mozzarella on hand for making pizzas.

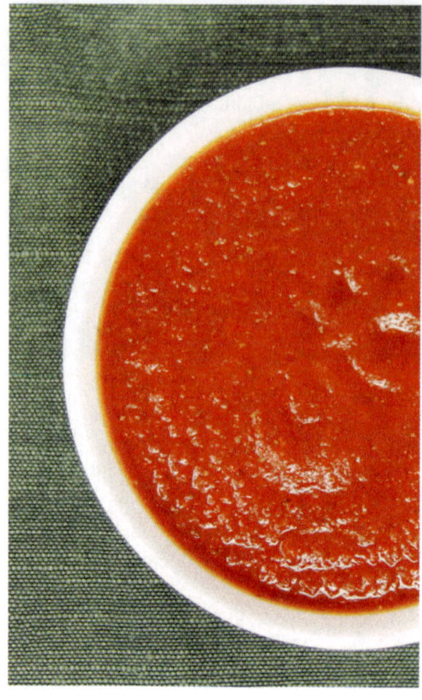

1 large onion, diced (about 1 ½ cups)

4 cloves garlic, pressed

2 (28 oz) cans of crushed tomatoes (or four 14-oz cans)

3 tbsp tomato paste, preferably low salt

1 tbsp Italian seasoning

1 tsp *maple syrup* (gradually reduce)

1 tbsp balsamic vinegar

½ cup chopped fresh basil

1 tsp *salt* (gradually reduce)

Pepper to taste

servings

Enough sauce for five 16-inch pizzas (about 2 ½ quarts)

equipment

Blender

1. Water sauté the onions until soft. Add the garlic and sauté for 30 more seconds.

2. Add the remaining ingredients and bring to a boil. Simmer for 15–20 minutes or until the sauce is thick.

3. Place in a blender and blend until smooth. Store in 5 equal portions in the refrigerator or freezer.

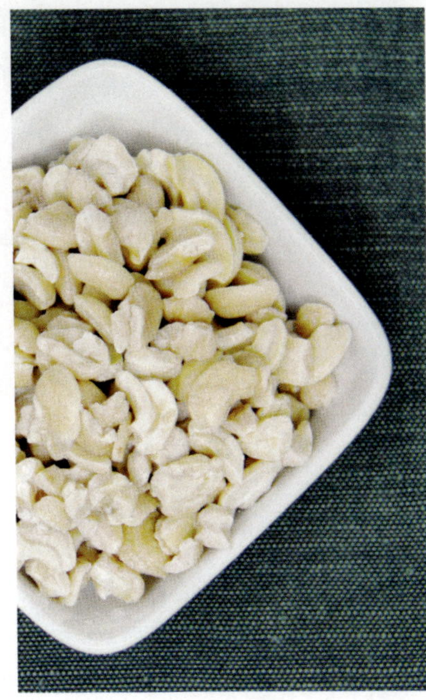

SOAKED CASHEWS

These are a main ingredient in WFPB cheeses, sour cream, and sweet creams. I always have a large resealable bag full of them in the freezer.

4 cups raw cashews

Water

servings

About 5 cups

1. Put the cashews in a large bowl and add water to a few inches above the cashews.

2. Let them soak 2–3 hours.

3. Drain, place in a resealable bag, and freeze.

SPICY BLACK BEANS

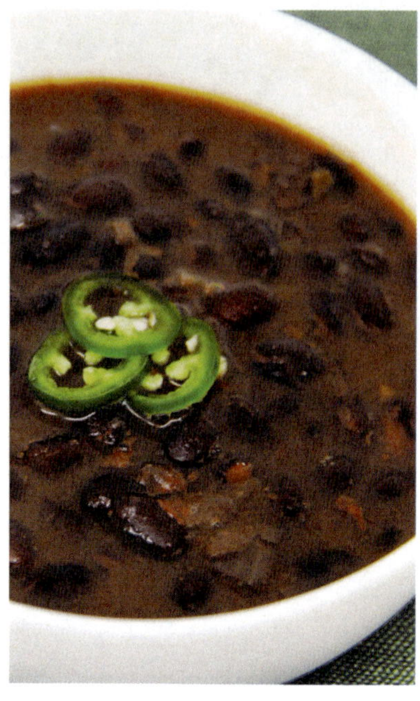

These beans are wonderful for bowls, Nachos (p 58), and Bean and Cheese Quesadillas (p 53), and are in the Black Bean and Corn Chili (p 40), and Nacho Salad (p 26). Making the beans yourself is cost effective and allows you to reduce the salt and adjust the spices to your taste. I freeze them in 16-oz portions, so I can use one jar to replace a can of beans in a recipe.

2 cups dried black beans

1 medium onion, diced (about 1 cup)

1 large clove garlic, pressed

2 tbsp finely minced jalapeño pepper (or to taste)

2 tbsp tomato paste, preferably low salt

2 tsp ground cumin

¼ tsp cayenne pepper (or to taste)

Pepper to taste

servings

About 6 cups

1. Soak the beans in cold water overnight at room temperature. Rinse in a strainer and set aside.

2. Water sauté the onions until soft. Add the garlic and jalapeño pepper and sauté for another 30 seconds.

3. Add the beans and remaining ingredients to the pot, add water to an inch above the beans and bring to a boil. Reduce heat and simmer 1–2 hours or until beans are tender but not mushy. Test them after 45 minutes and then every 10–15 minutes. Or cook them in a pressure cooker or Instant Pot to save time.

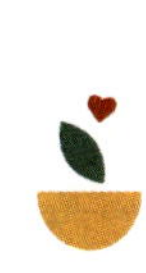

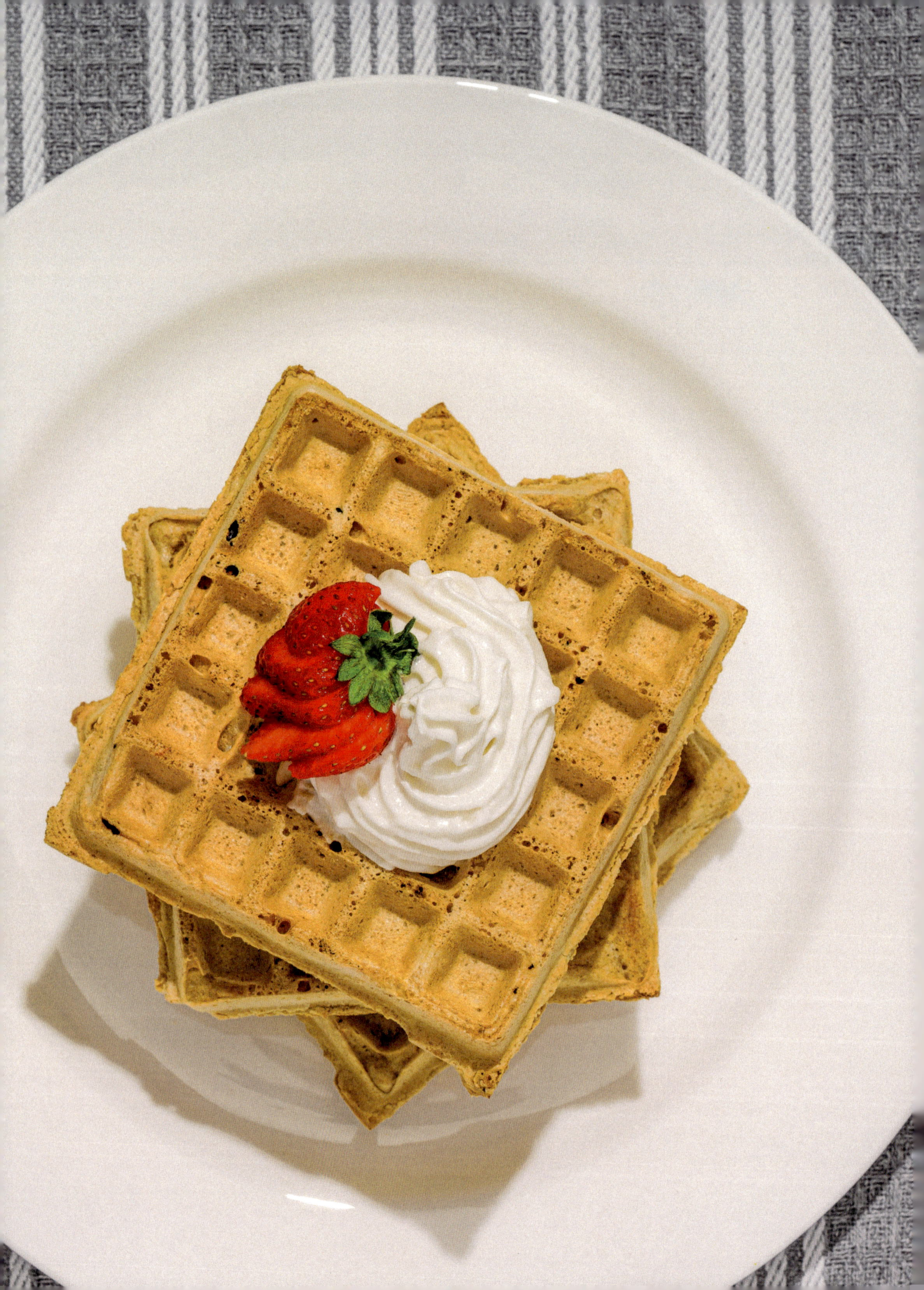

BREAKFAST FOODS

Our favorite breakfast foods are often the first to go when we transition to the whole food, plant based food plan, since they usually include eggs, dairy, or meat. After much experimenting, I have created some delicious WFPB versions of the forbidden favorites like cinnamon rolls, scones, waffles, pumpkin bread and more. It's so much fun to be able to make these again and enjoy them in good conscience.

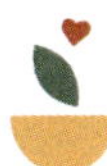

BLUEBERRY PANCAKES

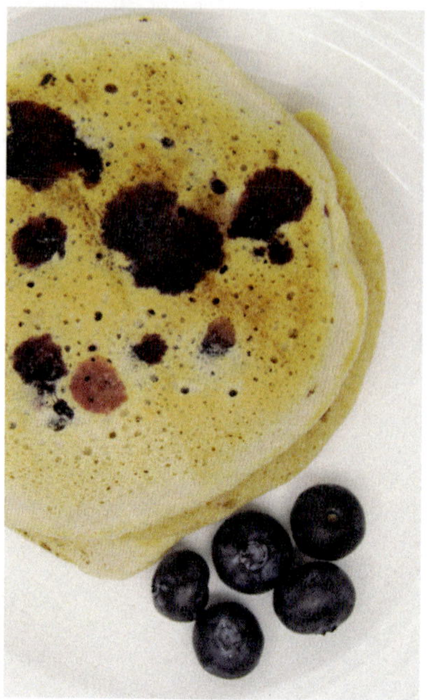

These blueberry pancakes have a light texture and taste a lot like classic breakfast restaurant pancakes. The reason they are so light is because they are made with the Waffle batter. I enjoy them with Vanilla Cashew Cream (p 140) and/or Fruit Purée (p 136). For a heartier pancake, try the Buckwheat Flax Pancakes (p 127).

1 cup unsweetened soy or other non-dairy milk

1 tbsp apple cider vinegar

1 tbsp *maple syrup* (gradually reduce)

1 tsp vanilla extract

1 cup whole wheat pastry flour

1 cup whole spelt flour (can be replaced with whole wheat flour)

2 tsp baking powder

½ tsp *salt* (gradually reduce)

½ cup aquafaba (water from cooking garbanzo beans or canned garbanzos)

½ cup water

1 ½ cups fresh or frozen blueberries, thawed

servings

About one dozen 4" pancakes

equipment

Nonstick griddle, hand mixer

1. Preheat a nonstick griddle to 375°F.

2. In a small bowl combine the non-dairy milk, apple cider vinegar, maple syrup, and vanilla and let stand 5 minutes.

3. In a large bowl, whisk together the flours, baking powder, and salt.

4. Add the non-dairy milk mixture and water to the dry ingredients and mix well. The batter will be quite thick.

5. Gently stir in the blueberries.

6. In a medium bowl, beat the aquafaba with a hand mixer until stiff peaks form.

7. Gently fold the whipped aquafaba into the batter.

8. Pour the batter onto the preheated griddle and cook for about 3 minutes on each side or until light golden brown on both sides and cooked through.

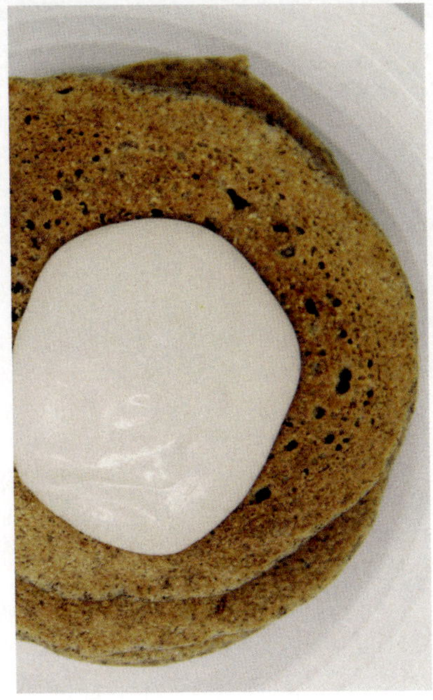

BUCKWHEAT FLAX PANCAKES

I thought my pancake eating days were over, especially because drenching anything in maple syrup is no longer a part of my food plan. Then there is the milk, butter, and refined flour in conventional pancakes. The non-dairy milk, apple cider vinegar, and whipped aquafaba in these pancakes make them light and moist, and the buckwheat flour and ground flax seed give them a hearty flavor. I love adding berries and walnuts to the batter. And instead of maple syrup, I top them with Vanilla Cashew Cream (p 140) and/or fresh fruit or a Fruit Purée (p 136). If you prefer a lighter pancake, Make the Blueberry Pancakes (p 126).

servings

12–14 (4") pancakes

equipment

Nonstick griddle, hand mixer

1 ½ cups unsweetened soy or other non-dairy milk

1 tbsp apple cider vinegar

1 tbsp *maple syrup* (gradually reduce)

2 tsp vanilla

¾ cup whole wheat pastry flour

¾ cup whole spelt flour (can be replaced with whole wheat flour)

½ cup buckwheat flour

2 tbsp fresh ground flax seeds

2 tsp baking powder

½ tsp *salt* (gradually reduce)

1–1 ½ cups berries (optional)

½ cup chopped walnuts (optional)

½ cup aquafaba

½ cup water or amount for desired texture

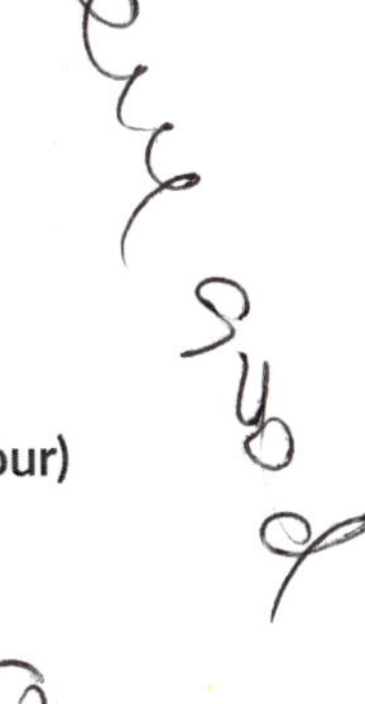

1. Preheat a nonstick griddle to 375°F.

2. In a small bowl, combine the non-dairy milk, vinegar, maple syrup, and vanilla and let stand 5 minutes.

3. In a large bowl, mix together dry ingredients.

4. Add the non-dairy milk mixture and berries or walnuts if using to the dry ingredients and stir until just mixed. Set aside.

5. In a medium bowl, beat the aquafaba with a hand mixer until stiff peaks form.

6. Gently fold the whipped aquafaba into the batter.

7. On the preheated griddle, cook on one side until bubbles appear and then flip and cook for a few more minutes on the other side until cooked through.

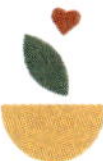

CHERRY ALMOND CHOCOLATE SCONES

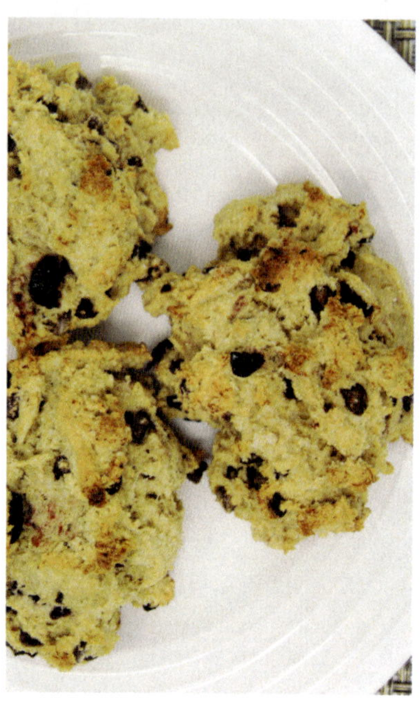

For years I looked for a WFPB scone recipe that was moist and flavorful. Finally, I discovered the power of soymilk curdled with apple cider vinegar for making baked goods moist and light. Enjoy these flavorful scones with Vanilla Almond Cashew Cream (p 140). These are also delicious made with chopped dried apricots instead of cherries.

1 cup unsweetened soy or other non-dairy milk

1 tbsp apple cider vinegar

2 tsp vanilla extract

2 tsp almond extract

1 tbsp *maple syrup*

1 ¾ cups whole wheat pastry flour

¾ cup blanched almond meal

1 tbsp baking powder

¼ tsp baking soda

½ tsp *salt* (gradually reduce)

⅓ cup chopped, dried tart cherries

¼ cup *mini vegan dark chocolate chips*

servings

About 12 scones

1. Preheat the oven to 450°F. Line a baking sheet with parchment paper.

2. In a medium bowl, mix the non-dairy milk, apple cider vinegar, vanilla and almond extracts, and maple syrup, and let stand 5 minutes.

3. In a large bowl, mix all dry ingredients together, including cherries and chocolate chips.

4. Add the non-dairy milk mixture to the dry ingredients and stir until just mixed.

5. Drop large dollops onto parchment paper on the baking sheet. Bake for 12–14 minutes or until golden brown on the bottom.

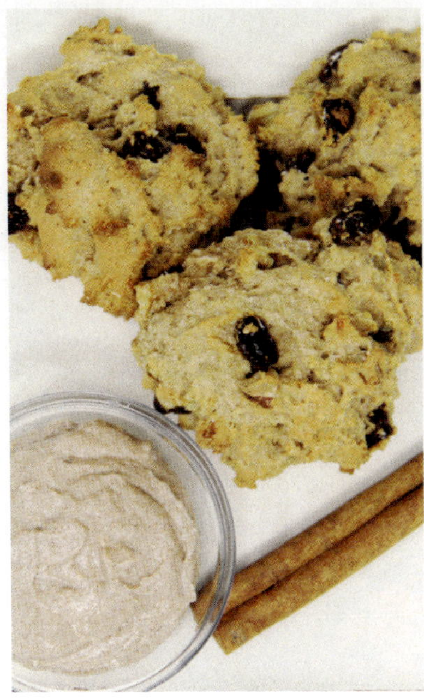

CINNAMON RAISIN SCONES

These scones are for cinnamon lovers. Serve with vanilla or date-sweetened cinnamon Cashew Cream (p 140). Try adding fresh fruit instead of dried fruit to the scones and experiment with different nuts and spices to develop your own favorite recipe.

servings

About 12 scones

1 cup unsweetened soy or other non-dairy milk

1 tbsp apple cider vinegar

2 tsp vanilla

1 tbsp *maple syrup*

1 ¾ cups whole wheat pastry flour

¾ cup blanched almond meal

1 tbsp baking powder

¼ tsp baking soda

1 tbsp cinnamon   *Increase*

½ tsp *salt* (gradually reduce)

½ cup raisins

½ cup walnuts (optional)

add almond flavoring and/or vanilla

1. Preheat the oven to 450°F. Line a baking sheet with parchment paper.

2. In a medium bowl, mix the non-dairy milk, apple cider vinegar, vanilla extract, and maple syrup, and let stand 5 minutes.

3. In a large bowl, mix all dry ingredients together, including raisins and walnuts.

4. Add the non-dairy milk mixture to the dry ingredients and stir until just mixed.

5. Drop large dollops onto parchment paper on the baking sheet. Bake for 12–14 minutes or until golden brown on the bottom.

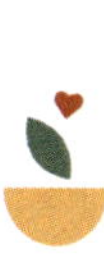

CINNAMON ROLLS

These are a classic breakfast or brunch treat. They are great with or without the frosting. You can also add cinnamon to the frosting if you're a big cinnamon lover.

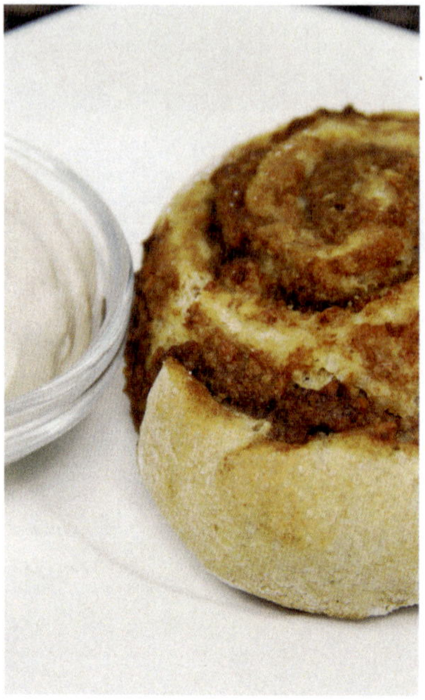

Dough

⅔ cup unsweetened soy or other non-dairy milk

2 tsp apple cider vinegar

½ cup water

1 ½ cups whole wheat pastry flour

1¼ cups whole spelt flour (can be replaced with whole wheat flour)

2 tsp yeast

½ tsp *salt*

1½ tbsp *maple syrup* (gradually reduce)

2 tsp vanilla extract

Filling

1 ¼ cup pitted, chopped medjool dates

½ cup boiling water

⅓ cup Soaked Cashews (p 121)

¼ cup water

1 tbsp cinnamon

2 tsp vanilla

½ cup ground walnuts or pecans

¼ cup raisins (optional)

½ cup coarsely chopped walnuts or pecans (optional)

Frosting

1 cup cashews

¼ cup water

2 tsp fresh lemon juice

1 tbsp vanilla

1 tbsp cinnamon (optional, for cinnamon lovers)

1½ tbsp *maple syrup* (eventually replace with ½ cup dates, chopped and soaked in ¼ cup boiling water)

Pinch of salt

Note: for a thicker frosting, you can blend the vanilla, cinnamon and dates with boiling water in a bullet-style blender and then mix with 1 cup of Fermented Cream Cheese (p 113).

servings

12–14 rolls

equipment

Bread machine (optional), bullet-style blender

Dough

1. In a small bowl, mix the non-dairy milk and the apple cider vinegar and let stand 5 minutes.

2. Put all ingredients including the non-dairy milk mixture in a bread machine and select the dough cycle.

If you do not have a bread machine, follow the instructions below.

1. In a small bowl, mix the non-dairy milk with the apple cider vinegar and let stand for 5 minutes.

2. In a large bowl, add the warm water to the yeast and let it rest for 5 minutes.

3. Add 1 cup of whole wheat pastry flour and the rest of the ingredients and mix on medium speed for 3 minutes.

4. Stir in 1 1/4 cups of whole spelt flour, mixing until the dough pulls away cleanly from the sides of the bowl.

5. On a floured surface, knead in up to 1/2 cup whole wheat pastry flour until the dough is smooth and elastic, about 10 minutes.

6. Place dough in a bowl, cover and let rise in a warm place until doubled in bulk, about 30–45 minutes.

7. Punch down and follow instructions below for assembling the rolls.

Filling

1. In a medium bowl, add the dates and boiling water. Cover and let stand 5 minutes.

2. Add the date mixture, soaked cashews, ¼ cup water, cinnamon, and vanilla to a bullet-style blender and blend until just a little bit grainy. The mixture should be very thick.

3. Stir in the ground walnuts or pecans. Reserve the raisins and chopped nuts for assembling the rolls.

Assembling the Rolls

1. When the dough is ready, place it on a large, lightly floured wooden cutting board or other clean, smooth surface, and roll out into a rectangle (about 14" x 20").

2. Spread the filling evenly over all of the dough with a spatula. Evenly sprinkle on the raisins and/or coarsely chopped nuts, if using.

3. Line a baking sheet with parchment paper.

4. With the long edge of the dough parallel to the edge of the counter closest to you, cut 1 ½ to 2-inch strips that are 14 inches long.

5. Carefully roll each strip of dough tightly into a spiral. You may need a silicon spatula or pastry cutter to gently lift the dough off the surface to roll it.

6. Place buns a few inches apart on the parchment paper on the baking sheet.

7. Cover the buns and set in a warm place to rise. I like to set my oven for 190°F for 2 minutes and then turn the oven off. I place the covered dough on the top oven rack and place a bowl with water that was just boiled on the lower rack. This makes the dough extra moist, light, and fluffy.

8. When the rolls have doubled in size, remove them and the bowl of water from the oven and preheat the oven to 425°F. Bake the rolls for 18–20 minutes or until slightly golden on the edges.

Frosting

1. If you are using dates instead of maple syrup, place the dates and boiling water in a small bowl, cover and let stand for 5 minutes.

2. Place all ingredients in a bullet-style blender and blend for 1–2 minutes or until smooth.

3. Spread the frosting over the buns once they have cooled or simply serve the frosting in a bowl along with the buns for anyone who wants some.

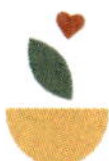

OATMEAL

Switching your breakfasts to oatmeal is a great first step in making the transition to a WFPB food plan. Before I started eating WFPB, I ate an egg for breakfast every morning. I really did not want to give up my eggs. But now I enjoy delicious oatmeal for breakfast most days. Top oatmeal with fresh berries, chopped walnuts, ground flax seed, hemp seed and unsweetened soy or other non-dairy milks. I cook oatmeal in large batches and store it in glass containers in the freezer and refrigerator.

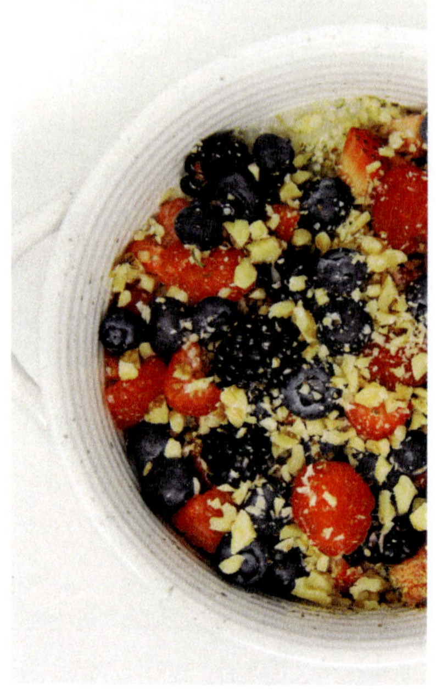

servings

8

4 cups steel cut oats (or 2 cups quick cooking steel cut and 2 cups rolled oats)

8 cups water (replace 2 cups of water with unsweetened soy or other non-dairy milk for a creamier texture)

1 large apple, cored, peeled, and chopped into small pieces (optional)

1–2 tbsp cinnamon (optional)

1. Bring the oats to a boil in the water. For regular steel cut oats, let cook for 30 minutes, then add apple pieces and cook for 5–10 more minutes. For quick cooking steel cut oats and rolled oats, add everything at once and let cook for 7–10 minutes.

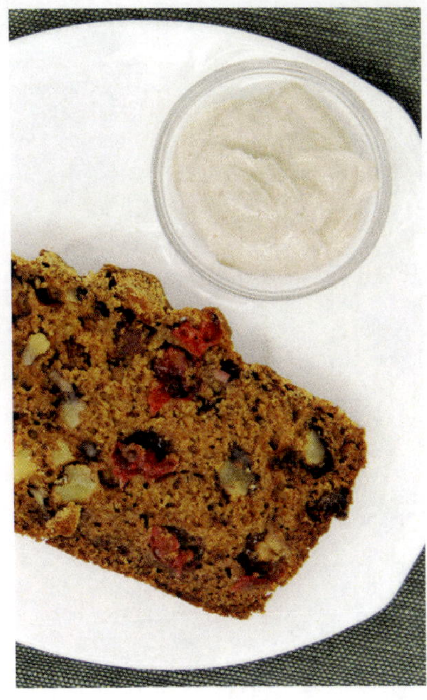

PUMPKIN CRANBERRY BREAD

This is another delicious way to eat pumpkin or kabocha squash. It is moist and tasty on its own, with date-sweetened Cream Cheese (p 112), or with vanilla, ginger, or nutmeg Cashew Cream (p 140).

servings

1 loaf

equipment

Bullet-style blender, loaf pan

⅓ cup pitted, chopped medjool dates

¼ cup boiling water

½ cup unsweetened soy or other non-dairy milk

1 tsp apple cider vinegar

¾ cup whole wheat flour

¾ cup whole spelt flour (can be replaced with whole wheat flour)

1 tsp baking soda

1 tsp baking powder

½ tsp *salt* (gradually reduce)

¼ tsp cinnamon

¼ tsp ground cloves

2 tsp ground ginger

¼ tsp ground nutmeg

1 cup coarsely chopped walnuts

1 cup coarsely chopped fresh or frozen cranberries

1 ½ cups pumpkin purée or steamed kabocha squash

1 tsp vanilla

2 tbsp *molasses*

1. Preheat oven to 350°F.

2. In a small bowl, add the dates and boiling water, cover and let stand 5 minutes.

3. In a medium bowl, combine the non-dairy milk, apple cider vinegar, vanilla, and molasses, and let stand for 5 minutes.

4. In a large bowl, mix all of the dry ingredients including the walnuts and cranberries.

5. Put the date mixture, pumpkin purée, and non-dairy milk mixture in a bullet-style blender and blend.

6. Mix the liquid ingredients into the dry ingredients.

7. Pour batter into a nonstick loaf pan and bake for an hour or until a knife comes out clean.

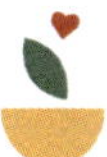

PUMPKIN NUGGETS

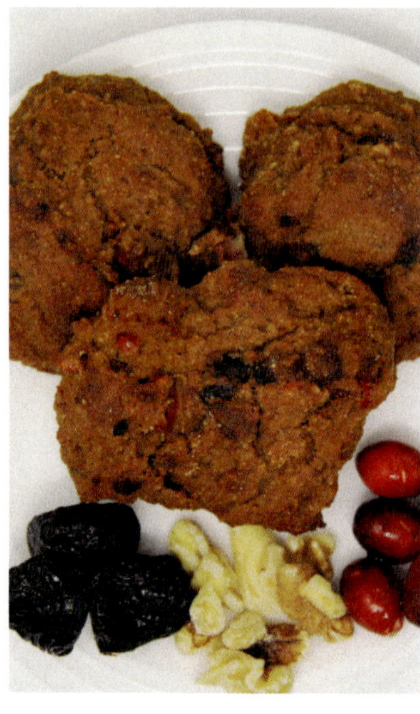

Even though these are easiest to make in the fall, they are a year-round favorite snack for me. I use fresh cranberries in the fall and frozen cranberries during the rest of the year. These nutrient and protein packed nuggets make a great treat on their own or toasted and topped with molasses Cashew Cream (p 140) with a cup of tea. They are perfect for taking on hikes, trips, or to work to keep you going.

1 cup unsweetened soy or other non-dairy milk

1 tbsp apple cider vinegar

2 tsp vanilla extract

2 tbsp *molasses*

⅓ cup quinoa flakes

¼ cup pitted, chopped medjool dates

2 tbsp boiling water

1 ¾ cups whole wheat pastry flour

¾ cup almond meal (use blanched for a lighter texture)

1 tbsp baking powder

¼ tsp baking soda

1 tbsp ginger

¼ tsp nutmeg

¼ tsp cinnamon

¼ tsp cloves

½ tsp *salt* (gradually reduce)

½ cup chopped walnuts

¾ cup chopped fresh or frozen cranberries

¾ cup chopped prunes or raisins

1 ½ cups pumpkin purée (fresh or canned) or steamed kabocha squash

servings

12–16 nuggets, depending on size

equipment

Bullet-style blender

1. In a medium bowl, mix the non-dairy milk, apple cider vinegar, vanilla extract, and molasses, and let stand 5 minutes. Add the quinoa flakes to the non-dairy milk mixture, stir with a fork, and let stand 10 minutes.

2. In a small bowl, add the dates and boiling water, cover and let stand 5 minutes.

3. Mix all other dry ingredients including the walnuts and fruit together in a bowl.

4. Preheat the oven to 450°F.

5. Put the pumpkin or kabocha squash, date mixture, and non-dairy milk mixture in a bullet-style blender and blend until smooth.

6. Add the pumpkin mixture to the dry ingredients. Stir until just mixed. Drop large dollops onto parchment paper on a baking sheet and bake for 12–15 minutes or until golden brown on the bottom.

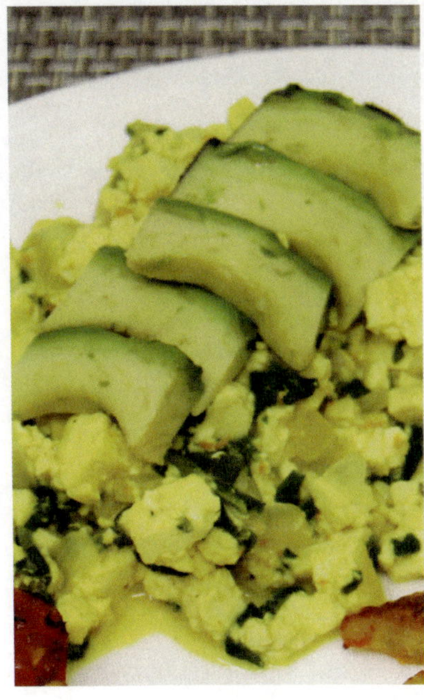

TOFU SCRAMBLE

This delicious scramble is a great way to transition away from eggs. Top with some black pepper and chopped chives or green onions and sliced avocado. Serve it with air fried potatoes or just enjoy with whole grain toast and a WFPB fruit spread.

2 tbsp Soaked Cashews (p 121)

1 tsp nutritional yeast

¼ tsp turmeric

⅔ cup water

Other seasonings or herbs of your choice (optional)

14 oz extra firm tofu

¼ cup diced onion

¾ cup small broccoli florets, sliced mushrooms, or other veggies of your choice (optional)

1 cup finely chopped baby spinach or other baby greens (optional)

Salt and pepper to taste (eventually omit salt)

1. Blend the cashews, nutritional yeast, turmeric, and water in a bullet-style blender until smooth.

2. Cut the tofu into small chunks.

3. In a medium glass storage container, add the tofu and cashew mixture and gently stir together. Put the lid on the container, shake the tofu around a little, and set aside.

4. Water sauté the onions and any other vegetables like broccoli or mushrooms (not including spinach or baby greens) on medium heat in a frying pan until they are soft. Pour the cooked veggies in a bowl and set aside.

5. In a medium frying pan, cook the tofu mixture for a minute, stirring, and then let simmer until most of the liquid has evaporated. Add the baby spinach or other baby greens and cooked veggies if you are using them and cook for another 2 minutes.

6. Remove from the heat and serve immediately.

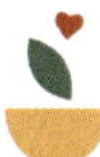

WAFFLES

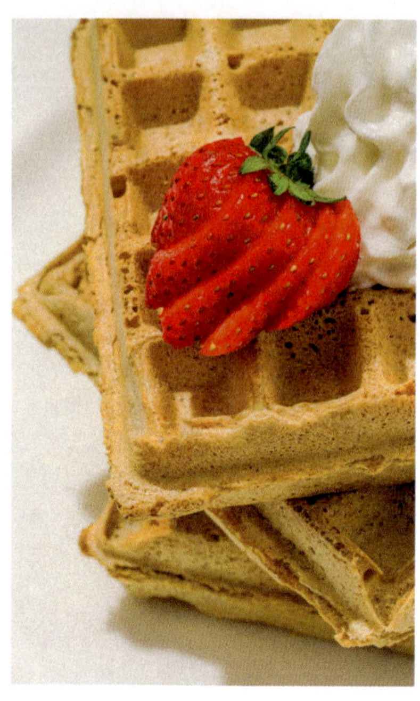

Waffles are one breakfast food that I had given up on ever being able to eat again on the WFPB food plan. I was thrilled when I discovered the wonders of aquafaba (garbanzo bean water) as a replacement for egg whites as well as the magic that soy milk mixed with apple cider vinegar works on making dough moist and fluffy. These crisp, fluffy waffles are a dream come true. I enjoy them with Vanilla Cashew Cream (p 140) and/or fresh fruit or Fruit Purée (see below). If you don't have a waffle maker, these make great pancakes, too! See Blueberry Pancakes (p 126).

servings

About 8 (4" x 4") waffles

equipment

Bullet-style blender, hand mixer, nonstick waffle iron

1 cup unsweetened soy or other non-dairy milk

1 tbsp apple cider vinegar

1 tbsp *maple syrup* (gradually reduce)

1 tsp vanilla extract

1 cup whole wheat pastry flour

1 cup whole spelt flour (can be replaced with whole wheat flour)

2 tsp baking powder

½ tsp *salt* (gradually reduce)

½ cup water

½ cup aquafaba (water from cooking garbanzo beans or canned garbanzos)

1. Preheat a nonstick waffle iron.
2. In a small bowl combine the non-dairy milk, apple cider vinegar, maple syrup, and vanilla and let stand 5 minutes.
3. In a large bowl, whisk together the flours, baking powder, and salt.
4. Add the non-dairy milk mixture and water to the dry ingredients and mix well. The batter will be quite thick.
5. In a medium bowl, beat the aquafaba with a hand mixer until stiff peaks form.
6. Gently fold the whipped aquafaba into the batter.
7. Pour the batter onto the hot waffle iron and cook according to the specifications of the waffle iron.

Fruit Purée

⅓–½ cup chopped, pitted medjool dates

½ cup boiling water

1 cup fresh or frozen berries

1. In a bullet-style blender cup, add the dates and boiling water, cover and let stand for five minutes.
2. Add the berries and blend all ingredients until smooth. Serve warm.

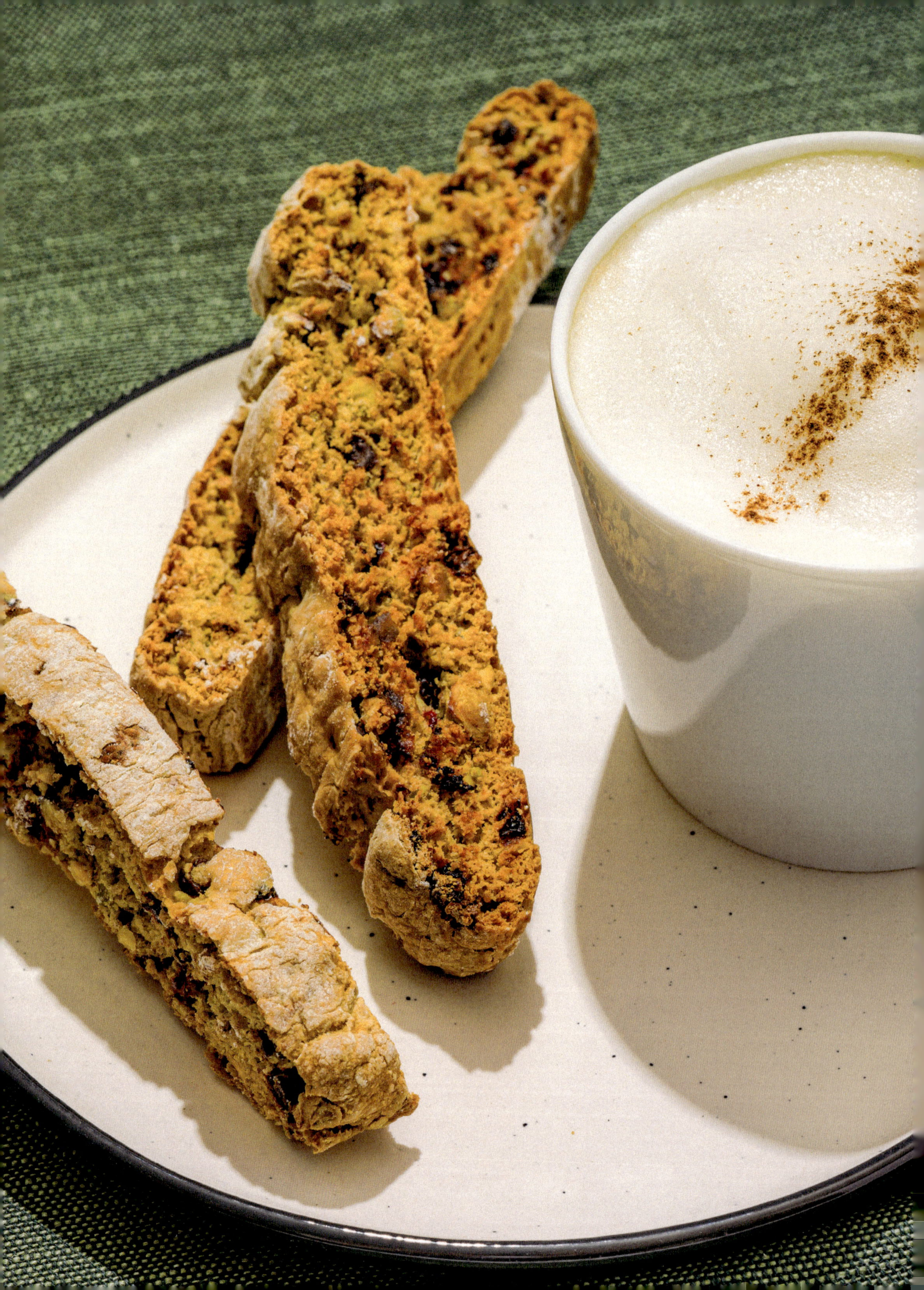

DESSERTS

Desserts can feel like another challenging part of transitioning to the WFPB food plan—and they needn't! We all have favorite birthday cakes and beloved holiday treats that we could not imagine those occasions without. And many of us just love having something yummy to munch on with coffee or tea. I was finally able to recreate my favorite sour cream chocolate birthday cake in WFPB form and there are many holiday cookies and other goodies I don't make any more. The good news is that I have also started some new food traditions that don't clog my arteries or make me gain weight, and that brings a lot of joy to my birthdays and the holidays. I encourage you to try WFPB versions of your favorite desserts where it is feasible and if it is not, then try something new. As your palate adapts, the really sweet desserts that we all used to eat will begin to taste too sweet and rich, and you will find more and more enjoyment in these healthier versions.

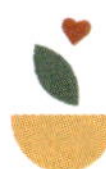

CASHEW CREAMS

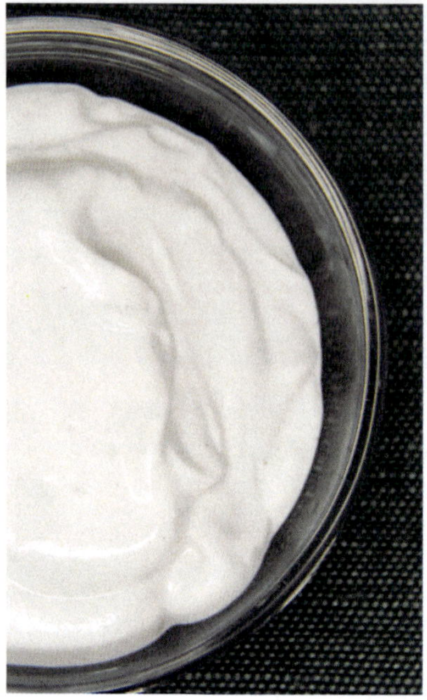

These cashew creams are a wonderful alternative to whipped cream. They are great with scones, waffles, and other baked goods—and there are a variety of flavors you can make to complement different dishes.

Maple Syrup Cream Base

¼–⅓ cup water (less water for a thicker cream)

1 tbsp *maple syrup*

1 cup Soaked Cashews (p 121)

Pinch *salt* (eventually omit)

1. Blend all ingredients, including the those for the flavor (see below), in a bullet-style blender for 2–3 minutes or until smooth.

Date Cream Base

½ cup pitted, chopped medjool dates

½ cup boiled water

1 cup Soaked Cashews (p 121)

Pinch *salt* (eventually omit)

1. In a small bowl, add the dates and boiling water, cover, and let stand 5 minutes.

2. Blend all ingredients, including the those for the flavor (see below), in a bullet-style blender for 2–3 minutes or until smooth.

servings

About 1 cup of cream

equipment

Bullet-style blender

Add any of the following to either of the cream bases to make these flavors:

Vanilla	Cinnamon	Nutmeg
2 tsp vanilla extract	2 tsp vanilla extract	½ tsp fresh ground nutmeg
	1 tbsp ground cinnamon	1 tsp vanilla

Vanilla Almond	Lemon Ginger	Molasses
2 tsp vanilla extract	2 tbsp grated lemon zest	1 tbsp molasses (use Maple Syrup Cream Base and leave out the maple syrup)
2 tsp almond extract	1 tsp grated fresh ginger	

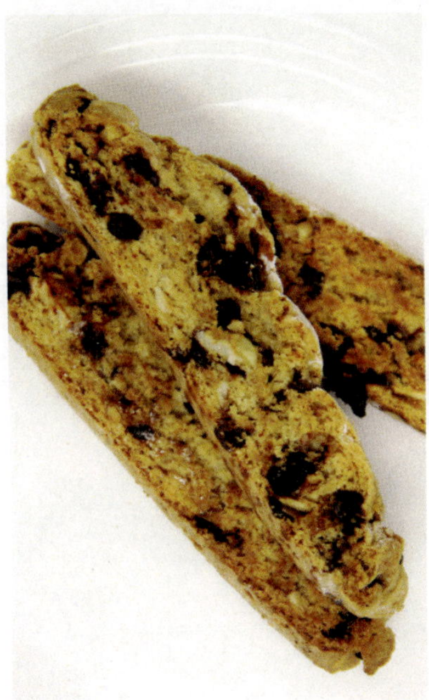

CHERRY ALMOND CHOCOLATE BISCOTTI

servings

25–30 biscotti, depending on the thickness

I love dunking these crisp biscotti in golden milk, tea, or coffee. The cherries are tart and chewy and the nuts are crisp. In an airtight container at room temperature, they will last 7–10 days.

1 cup unsweetened soy or other non-dairy milk

1 tbsp apple cider vinegar

2 tsp vanilla extract

2 tsp almond extract

2–3 tbsp *maple syrup*

1 ¾ cups whole wheat pastry flour

½ cup blanched almond meal

¼ cup *tapioca flour* (optional for a lighter texture or replace with ¼ cup whole wheat pastry flour)

2 tsp baking powder

¼ tsp baking soda

½ tsp *salt* (gradually reduce)

⅓ cup finely chopped, dried tart cherries

⅓ cup slivered or finely chopped almonds

¼ cup *mini vegan dark or semisweet chocolate chips*

1. Preheat the oven to 450°F. Line a baking sheet with parchment paper.

2. In a medium bowl, add the non-dairy milk, apple cider vinegar, vanilla and almond extracts, and maple syrup, and let stand 5 minutes.

3. In a large bowl, mix all dry ingredients together, including cherries, almonds, and chocolate chips.

4. Add the non-dairy milk mixture to the dry ingredients, and stir until just mixed.

5. Use tapioca or whole wheat pastry flour on your hands and the dough as you shape it into two loaves about 1 inch thick by 4 inches wide by 8 inches long on the parchment-lined baking sheet.

6. Bake the two loaves for 15 minutes.

7. Remove from the oven and turn the temperature down to 400°F. Put the warm loaves on a cutting board and let sit for 1–2 minutes.

8. Cut ½ inch–wide slices that are the width of the loaf (not the length). Traditional biscotti are cut holding the knife at a 30° angle to the short edge of the loaf. However, I like to cut them straight so that all of the biscotti are the same size. It helps to use a serrated bread knife and gently cut into the top of the loaf, then press straight down. Otherwise, you can tear the biscotti by sawing the bread knife back and forth across the dough.

9. Lay the slices flat on the baking sheet and bake for 6 minutes, then flip the cookies and bake another 6 minutes.

10. Turn the oven off and leave the biscotti in the oven for another 20–30 minutes to dry out and get crisp.

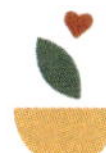

CHERRY PISTACHIO CHOCOLATE BISCOTTI

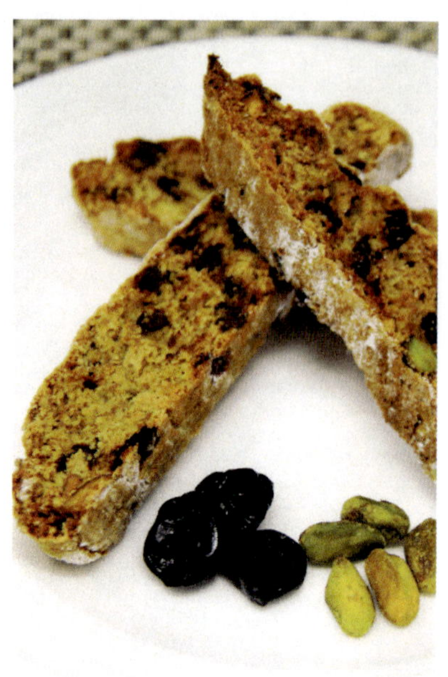

While both flavors of biscotti are delicious, these are my favorite, because the pistachios have a great flavor and make the biscotti extra crisp. Try making these with your own favorite ingredients!

1 cup unsweetened soy or other non-dairy milk

1 tbsp apple cider vinegar

2 tsp vanilla extract

1 tbsp pistachio extract

2–3 tbsp *maple syrup*

1 ¾ cups whole wheat pastry flour

¼ cup *tapioca flour* (optional for a lighter texture, or you can replace with ¼ cup more whole wheat pastry flour)

½ cup ground raw pistachios

2 tsp baking powder

¼ tsp baking soda

½ tsp *salt* (gradually reduce)

⅓ cup dried tart cherries

½ cup coarsely chopped pistachios

¼ cup *mini vegan dark or semisweet chocolate chips*

servings

> 25–30 biscotti, depending on the thickness

1. Preheat oven to 450°F. Line a baking sheet with parchment paper.

2. In a medium bowl, mix the non-dairy milk, apple cider vinegar, vanilla and pistachio extracts, and maple syrup, and let stand 5 minutes.

3. Mix all dry ingredients together, including the cherries, pistachios, and chocolate chips in a bowl.

4. Add the non-dairy milk mixture to the dry ingredients, and stir until just mixed.

5. Use tapioca or whole wheat pastry flour on your hands and the dough as you shape it into two loaves about 1 inch thick by 4 inches wide by 8 inches long on the parchment-lined baking sheet.

6. Bake the two loaves for 15 minutes.

7. Remove from the oven and turn the temperature down to 400°F. Put the warm loaves on a cutting board and let sit for 1–2 minutes.

8. Cut ½ inch–wide slices that are the width of the loaf (not the length). Traditional biscotti are cut holding the knife at a 30° angle to the short edge of the loaf. However, I like to cut them straight so that all of the biscotti are the same size. Also, it helps to use a bread knife and gently cut into the top of the loaf, then press straight down. Otherwise, you can tear the biscotti by sawing the bread knife back and forth across the dough.

9. Lay the slices flat on the baking sheet and bake for 6 minutes, then flip the cookies and bake another 6 minutes.

10. Turn the oven off and leave the biscotti in the oven for another 20–30 minutes to dry out and become crisp.

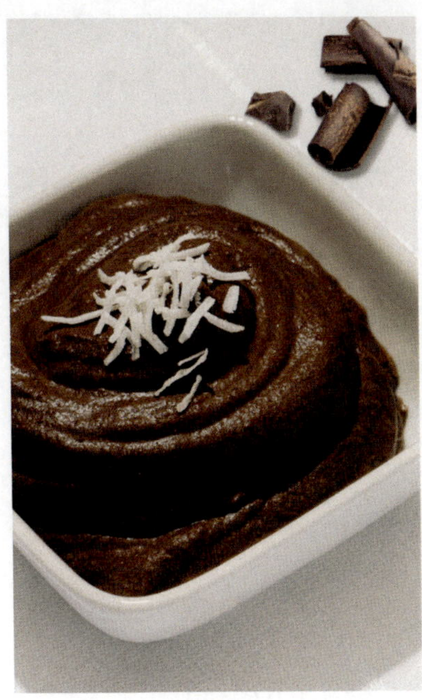

CHOCOLATE PUDDING

This creamy pudding hits the spot, especially in the early months of transitioning to WFPB eating. Try topping it with coconut flakes or vanilla Cashew Cream (p 140). This pudding is very rich.

⅓ cup pitted, chopped medjool dates

¼ cup boiling water

1 cup Soaked Cashews (p 121)

3 tbsp unsweetened cocoa powder

2 tsp vanilla extract

Pinch of salt

Water as needed for consistency

Add any of the following to the pudding to make these flavors:

Chocolate Almond
2 tsp almond extract

Chocolate Coconut
2 tbsp unsweetened coconut flakes

Chocolate Cherry
2 tbsp tart cherry concentrate

1. In a small bowl, add the dates and boiling water, cover, and let stand for 5 minutes.

2. Add all ingredients, including the those for the flavors to a bullet-style blender and blend for 3 minutes or until smooth and creamy. Add water 1 tablespoon at a time until the pudding is the desired consistency.

servings

4 small servings

equipment

Bullet-style blender

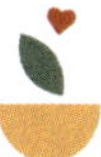

CHOCOLATE-COVERED CHERRY FROZEN CREAM

This decadent dessert is a great alternative to real ice cream. Lots of flavor, no guilt!

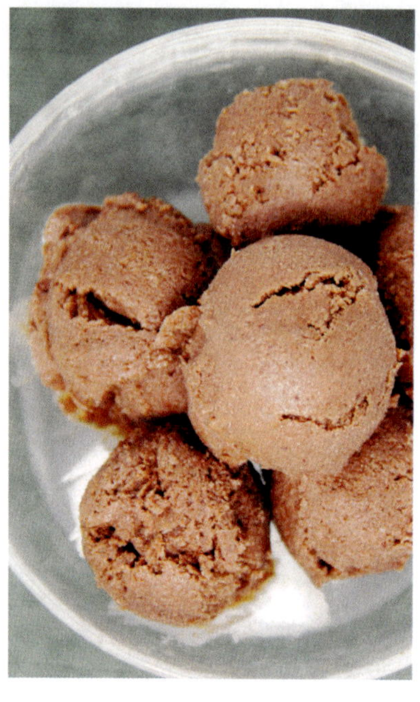

1 cup pitted, chopped medjool dates

½ cup boiling water

¼ cup unsweetened cocoa powder

½ cup Soaked Cashews (p 121)

1¼ cups frozen cherries

¼ cup unsweetened soy or other non-dairy milk

2 tsp vanilla extract

1 tbsp tart cherry concentrate (optional for more flavor and antioxidants)

servings

About 2 cups

equipment

Bullet-style blender

1. In a medium bowl, add the dates and boiling water, cover, and let stand for 5 minutes.

2. Blend all ingredients in a bullet-style blender for 2 minutes or until smooth.

3. Place in a sealed glass container in the freezer.

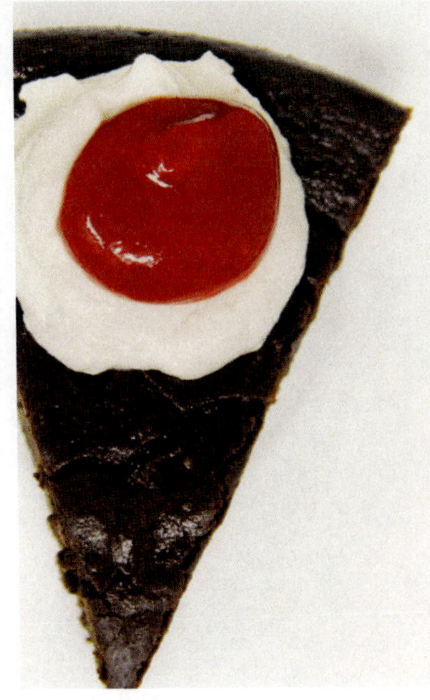

This is the cake I baked for so many family birthday celebrations over the years. After years of going without it, I was thrilled when I finally came up with a WFPB version using Special Sour Cream (see below) and aquafaba (garbanzo bean water). I frost it with vanilla Cashew Cream (p 140) and drizzle it with Raspberry Purée (see below).

This is a very rich and dense cake, so I make it in an 8" springform pan. It is about 2" thick.

servings

6–8

equipment

Bullet-style blender

Special Sour Cream

Makes about 1 cup

1 cup Soaked Cashews (p 121)

⅓ cup fresh lemon juice

¼ tsp *salt*

¼ cup water

1. Add all ingredients to a bullet-style blender. Blend on high for 2–3 minutes or until smooth and creamy.

Raspberry Purée

⅓–½ cup chopped, pitted medjool dates

½ cup boiling water

1 cup frozen raspberries

1. In a bullet blender cup, add the dates and boiling water, cover and let stand for five minutes.

2. Add the berries and blend all ingredients until smooth. Serve cool.

---

1 ¼ cups pitted, chopped medjool dates

½ cup boiling water

1 cup unsweetened soy or other non-dairy milk

1 tbsp apple cider vinegar

2 tsp vanilla extract

2 tbsp maple syrup

1 cup whole wheat pastry flour

½ cup blanched almond flour

2 tsp baking powder

1 tsp baking soda

¼ tsp *salt*

¾ cup unsweetened cocoa powder

½ cup Special Sour Cream (see below)

½ cup aquafaba

1. Preheat the oven to 350°F.

2. In a medium bowl, add the dates and boiling water, cover, and let stand 5 minutes.

3. In a small bowl, add the non-dairy milk, apple cider vinegar, vanilla extract, and maple syrup, and let stand 5 minutes.

4. In a large bowl, combine flours, baking powder, baking soda, salt, and cocoa powder, and whisk together.

5. In a bullet-style blender, add the date and non-dairy milk mixture, and blend until smooth.

6. Pour the liquid from the bullet-style blender and the sour cream into the bowl with the dry ingredients and mix together with a hand mixer.

7. In a separate bowl, whip the aquafaba until it forms stiff peaks. Then fold into the chocolate batter.

8. Pour into a nonstick 8-inch round cake pan (preferably springform) and bake for 50–60 minutes or until a knife comes out mostly clean.

9. Frost with vanilla cashew cream and drizzle with raspberry purée.

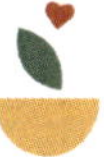

PUMPKIN PECAN TARTLETS

These creamy pumpkin custard tartlets, topped with toasted pecans and dates, are a perfect holiday dessert. I like to keep some in the freezer in case someone comes over for tea.

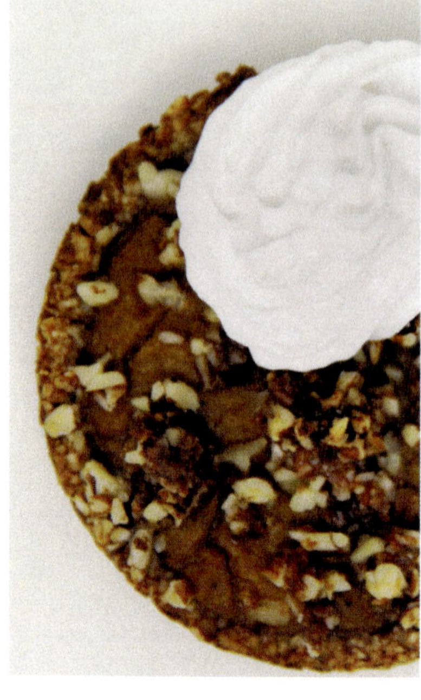

Crust

½ cup pitted, chopped medjool dates

½ cup boiling water

1 cup rolled oats (or 1 cup oat flour)

1 cup raw pecans

Pinch of salt

Topping

½ cup pecans

¼ cup pitted, chopped medjool dates

Filling

1 ½ cups steamed kabocha squash or 1 can (15 oz) pumpkin purée

1½ cups unsweetened soy or other non-dairy milk

2 tbsp *tapioca flour*

1 tsp vanilla extract

1 ½ tsp pumpkin pie spice blend (or replace with ½ tsp cinnamon, ½ tsp ginger, ¼ tsp nutmeg, ¼ tsp allspice, and ¼ tsp cloves)

½ teaspoon *salt* (gradually reduce)

⅔ cup pitted, chopped medjool dates (use more for a sweeter custard)

Crust

1. In a small bowl, add the dates and boiling water, cover, and let stand for 5 minutes, then drain.

2. Blend the oats in a food processor or blender until they form a fine flour (or just add oat flour to the food processor). Add the pecans and salt and blend until smooth. Add the drained dates and blend until it is a sticky dough.

3. Roll balls of about 1 ½ tbsp of the mixture and press flat in the cups of a nonstick muffin top tin (a regular nonstick muffin tin can be used as well). The dough should come up the side of the muffin cup ¼–½ inch. Set aside.

Filling

1. Add all ingredients to a bullet-style blender and blend until smooth.

2. Pour into a medium saucepan and bring to a gentle boil over medium heat, stirring constantly. Remove from the heat as soon as the custard has thickened. Set aside.

Topping

1. In a very small food processor or blender, blend the pecans and dates until they are in small pieces but not a fine meal.

Assembly

1. Preheat the oven to 350°F.

2. Pour ¼ cup of the filling into each tartlet crust.

3. Sprinkle a small amount of the topping onto each tartlet.

4. Bake for 15–18 minutes or until the crust and topping are golden.

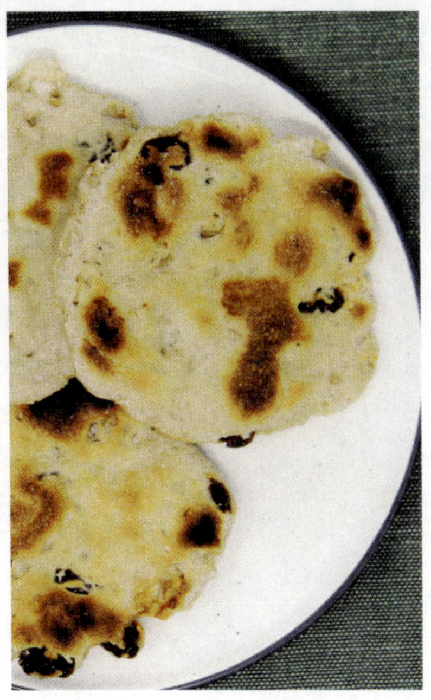

RAISIN WALNUT FLATBREADS

These not very sweet, chewy biscuits are delicious dipped in golden milk or tea. As your tastes change, you may find, like I did, that the sweetness of the raisins is enough to satisfy the desire for a cookie or dessert. Make a big batch and freeze them, and reheat them in the toaster. Add your own favorite dried fruits, nuts, and spices.

¼ cup unsweetened soy or other non-dairy milk

1½ tsp apple cider vinegar

1 cup whole wheat flour

¾ cups whole spelt flour (can be replaced with whole wheat flour)

1 ½ tsp active dry yeast

½ cup warm water

½ tsp *maple syrup*

½ tsp *salt*

½ cup chopped walnuts

½ cup raisins

servings

10–12 small rounds

equipment

Bread machine (optional), hand mixer, nonstick griddle

1. In a small bowl, combine non-dairy milk and apple cider vinegar, and let stand 5 minutes.

2. Add all ingredients except the walnuts and raisins to the bread machine and select the dough setting.

If you do not have a bread machine, follow the instructions below.

1. *In a small bowl, mix the non-dairy milk with the apple cider vinegar and let stand for 5 minutes.*

2. *In a large bowl, add the warm water to the yeast and let it rest for 5 minutes.*

3. *Add ¾ cup of whole spelt flour and the rest of the ingredients and mix on medium speed for 3 minutes.*

4. *Stir in ¾ cup of whole wheat pastry flour, mixing until the dough pulls away cleanly from the sides of the bowl.*

5. *On a floured surface, knead in up to ¼ cup whole wheat pastry flour until the dough is smooth and elastic, about 10 minutes.*

6. *Place dough in a bowl, cover and let rise in a warm place until doubled in bulk, about 30–45 minutes.*

7. *Punch down and follow instructions below for assembling the rolls.*

3. When the dough is ready, preheat a nonstick griddle to 400°F.

4. On a floured board, knead the raisins and walnuts into the dough.

5. Roll the dough into 1 ½–inch balls and flatten onto the griddle. Cook 2–4 minutes on each side or until they have some golden brown spots.

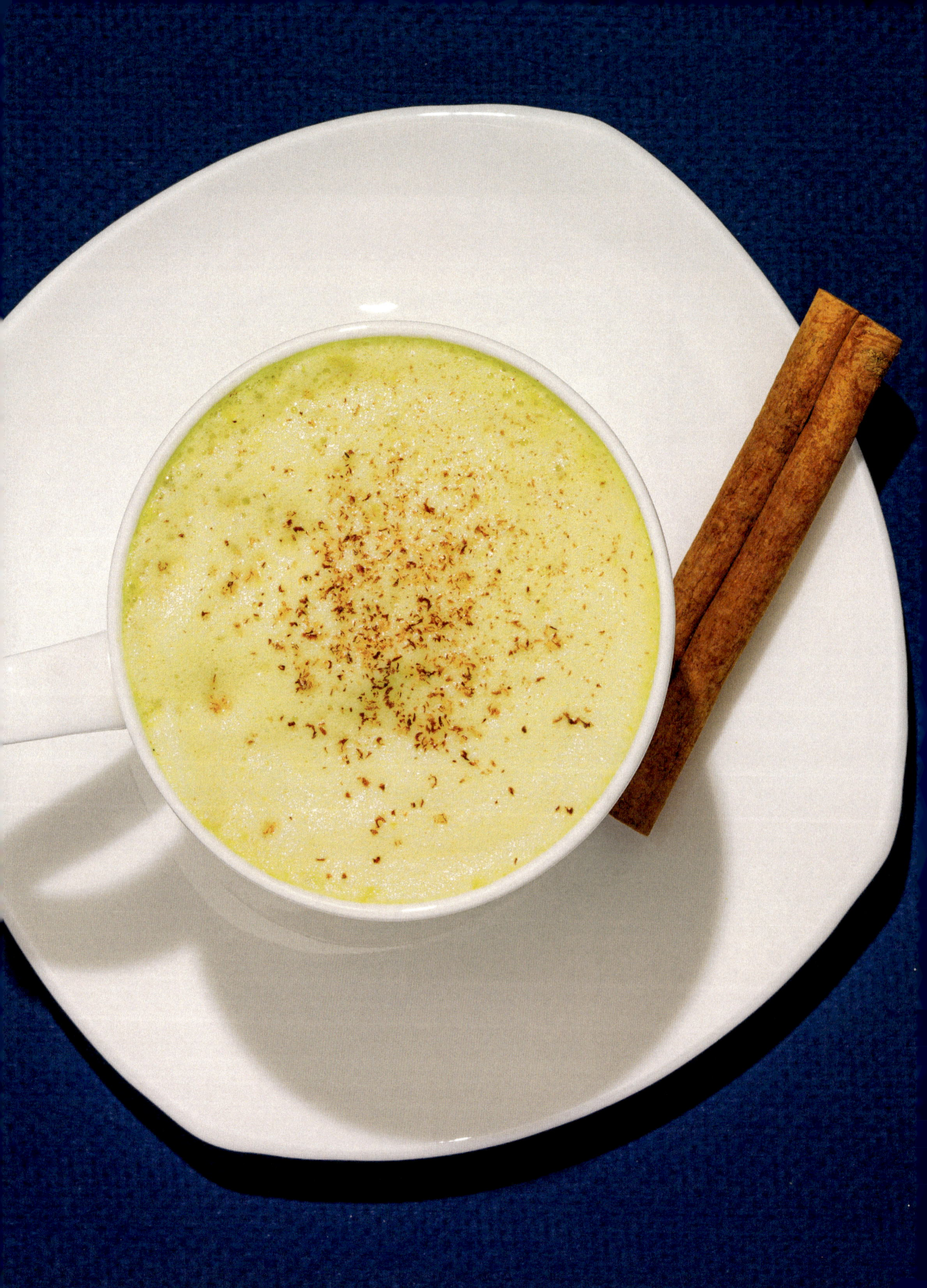

DRINKS

So many commercially available drinks are loaded with calories, sugar, artificial flavors and sweeteners, and many coffee drinks are also high in fat. Moving away from these types of beverages is an important part of transitioning to the WFPB food plan.

Even just infusing water with mint, cucumber, lemon, or other herbs and fruits can make a surprisingly flavorful and refreshing drink. When I think about having a cocktail or a glass of wine, I make one of the sparklers to have with my meal instead. I am always glad I made that choice.

Many people want to know if coffee can be a part of a WFPB food plan. Although it is acidic, studies show that coffee is high in antioxidants and can be beneficial for brain function and mood. However, some doctors recommend against drinking coffee or other caffeinated beverages because they can trigger the pleasure trap reaction, which can lead to cravings. Coffee or tea with a little maple syrup and non-dairy milk can be a part of your transitional food plan. Green tea is also very high in antioxidants and most doctors recommend drinking it, even though it has a little caffeine.

It's important not to let the prospect of giving up caffeinated drinks stop you from going WFPB. I personally drink a small amount of caffeinated drinks, and it's up to you to decide what works best for your body.

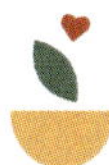

COMFORT TEA

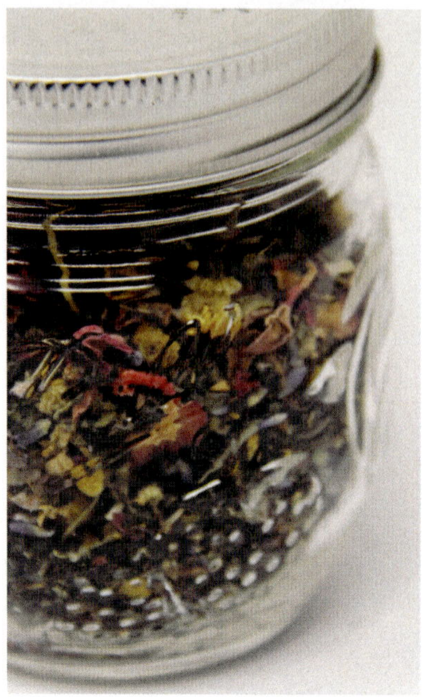

This caffeine free tea is a wonderful blend for nourishing and relaxing the body. Traditionally, nettles have been used to help the urinary tract and fight inflammation, chamomile, lavender, and peppermint to aid digestion and help reduce stress, and rose petals are thought to be good for the skin. Drink it at night to help you get a good night's sleep. A jar of this tea also makes a great handmade gift!

These herbs can be purchased at herb stores, some health food stores, and online.

Ingredients for tea blend (to make a jar of tea)

½ cup dried nettles

½ cup dried chamomile

¾ cup dried, organic, food grade rose petals

¼ cup dried peppermint

2 tbsp dried lavender

servings

About 2 cups of dried tea blend or 16 cups of tea

equipment

Tea leaf ball

1. Thoroughly combine all of the ingredients and keep in a tightly-closed mason jar.

2. For an individual cup, put 2 tsp in a tea leaf ball, add boiling water, and let steep for 4–6 minutes or to taste. Use 1 ½ tbsp for an 18-oz pot.

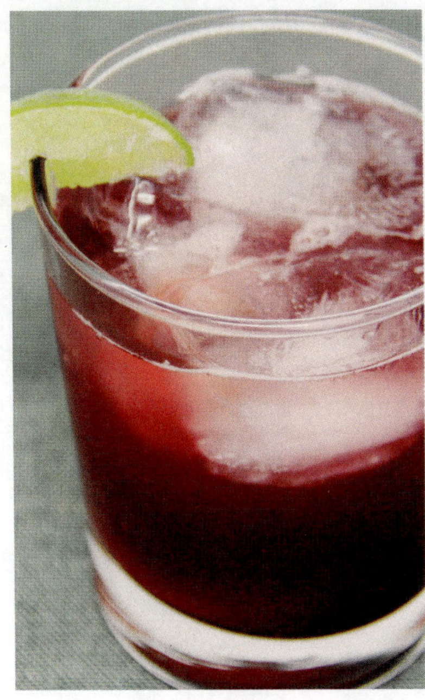

servings

1 drink

CRANBERRY LIME SPARKLER

This is a simple and refreshing alternative to a cocktail. I like to order it if I am with people who are having alcoholic drinks.

Ice (optional)

¾ cup sparkling water

Juice of 1 lime slice or to taste

Splash of cranberry juice (1–2 tbsp)

1. Add all ingredients to a glass of ice (if using). Garnish with a lime slice.

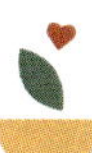

LOVEJOY GOLDEN MILK

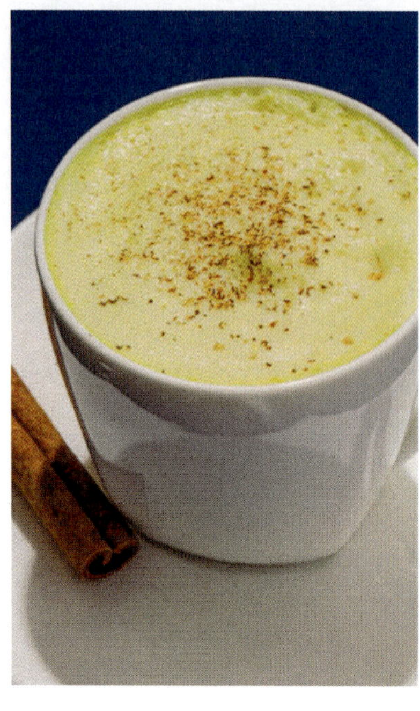

This is one of my most beloved comfort drinks. The herbs and spices in golden milk are used in many cultures to settle the stomach and calm the nerves, in addition to being high in antioxidants and other nutrients. It is wonderful for dipping biscotti in or for just sipping from a mug by the fire. Try frothing it in a milk frother and topping with fresh, grated nutmeg.

These herbs and spices can all be purchased at a grocery or health food store.

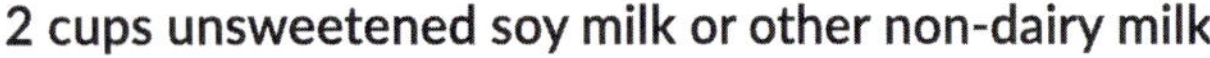

servings

2

equipment

Milk frother (optional)

2 cups unsweetened soy milk or other non-dairy milk

¼ cup water

10 whole cardamom pods, bruised

10 whole cloves

2 cinnamon sticks chopped/broken into smaller pieces

3 black peppercorns coarsely ground in a mortar and pestle or pepper grinder

1 tsp grated fresh ginger

1 tsp grated fresh turmeric

1 inch of fresh vanilla bean or 1 tsp vanilla extract

1 tbsp *maple syrup* (gradually reduce)

1. Pour non-dairy milk and water in a medium saucepan.

2. Add everything except the vanilla extract (if you are using a vanilla bean, add it now) and the maple syrup and bring to a boil. Watch the pot closely as the mixture can boil over easily. Reduce heat and simmer for only 5 minutes.

3. Pour the liquid through a strainer, stir in the vanilla extract and maple syrup, froth, if desired, and serve.

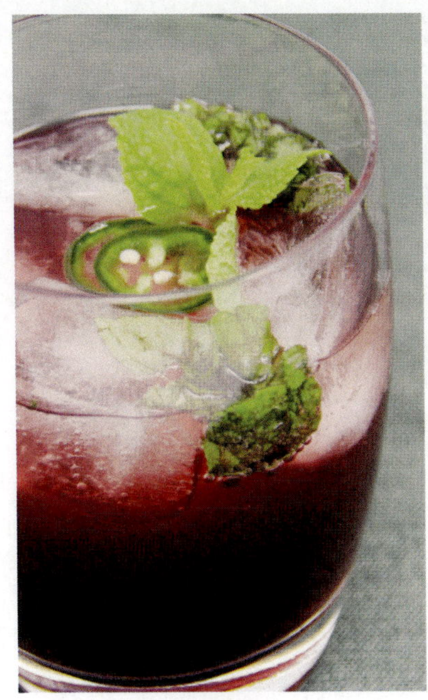

POMEGRANATE MINT SPARKLER

This is my favorite "cocktail." I love the tart pomegranate with the tangy ginger kombucha and the smooth mint. The jalapeño slices give it a gentle bite.

Kombucha is a fermented, probiotic tea that is thought to be beneficial for digestive health. It can be purchased in most grocery stores and in health food stores. Try to avoid brands with added sugar or artificial flavorings.

I use a small mortar and pestle to muddle the mint. You can also buy a muddler (to muddle the mint in the glass) at cooking supply stores or online.

2 tsp muddled mint

¼ cup pure pomegranate juice (no sugar added)

¼ cup ginger kombucha

½ cup sparkling water

1–2 slices jalapeño pepper (optional)

Ice (optional)

1. Place the muddled mint in the bottom of the glass and add the jalapeño slices (if using).

2. Pour the other ingredients into the glass. Add ice as needed.

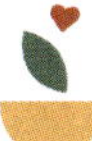

ROSE TEA LATTE

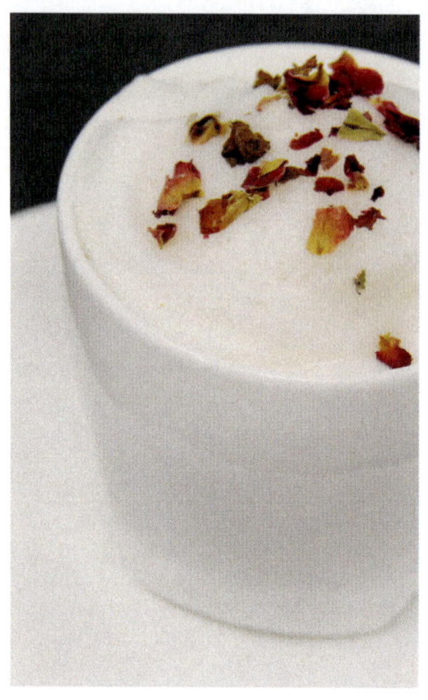

This is a nice alternative to coffee and is great with biscotti and scones.

The rose petals can be purchased at herb stores, some health food stores, and online.

Tea Blend

½ cup loose, black tea leaves of your choice (I use Assam)

1 cup organic, food grade, dried rose petals

Thoroughly mix black tea leaves with the rose petals and place in a tightly-sealed mason jar.

Latte

2–3 tsp rose tea blend from the jar

¼ cup unsweetened soy milk or other non-dairy milk

¼ tsp vanilla extract

½ tsp *maple syrup or honey* (gradually reduce)

1. For an individual latte, put 2 tsp of the tea mixture in a tea ball, add boiling water, and let steep for two minutes or more as desired.

2. Remove the tea ball from the cup and add ¼ tsp maple syrup or honey to the tea.

3. In a milk frother, add non-dairy milk, ¼ tsp vanilla extract, and remaining ¼ tsp maple syrup or honey and froth.

4. Pour the frothy milk into the tea and enjoy.

servings

1½ cups of dried tea blend or 20–24 cups of tea

equipment

Milk frother, tea leaf ball

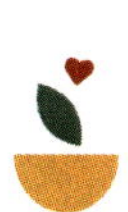

SAMPLE MEAL PLAN

Here are some meal plan ideas. It's important to cook the foods in large batches and freeze some so that, after a few weeks, you will have a variety of food available to you. That being said, you don't need to have much variety in your diet if you don't want to. I eat oatmeal almost every day for breakfast. If I have pancakes, waffles, or scones, I have them for snacks or desserts. You can eat anything you want anytime of day. Just remember to add salad, beans, and greens as much as possible. Doctors recommend eating at least a handful of cooked leafy greens every day. I like water sautéing them with shallots or onions.

The longer you are on the food plan, the more you will want to focus on eating bowls, salads, soups, chilis, and curries as these are the highest nutrient foods in the cookbook. And then eventually you may be ready to try a stricter WFPB food plan. Relax, there is no rush. You are already making the transition and will begin to experience the benefits very quickly.

	MONDAY	TUESDAY	WEDNESDAY
Breakfast	Oatmeal w/ berries, ground flax seed, hempseed and chopped walnuts w/ non-dairy milk Tea or coffee w/ non-dairy milk	Buckwheat flax pancakes w/ fruit purée Tea or coffee w/ non-dairy milk	Mushroom/spinach tofu scramble w/ sliced avocados WFPB toast w/ fruit purée Tea or coffee w/ non-dairy milk
Snack	Scone with cashew cream and tea	Avocado toast	Pumpkin nugget and green tea
Lunch	Falafel w/ naan bread Salad	Spaghetti w/ sautéed greens and roasted garlic bread	Quesadilla w/ taco slaw Sliced fruit and biscotti
Snack	Hummus veggie toast	Crackers and/or veggies and hummus	Baked potato w/ sour cream and green onions
Dinner	Southwestern bowl	Southwestern kale and white bean soup w/ green onion cornbread biscuit Salad	Curry w/ naan bread Salad
Snack	Sliced apple/ pumpkin seeds	Golden milk and biscotti	Cinnamon roll and comfort tea

THURSDAY	FRIDAY	SATURDAY	SUNDAY
Oatmeal w/ berries, ground flax seed, hempseed and chopped walnuts w/ non-dairy milk Tea or coffee w/ non-dairy milk	Blueberry pancakes w/ vanilla cream and blueberry purée Tea or coffee w/ non-dairy milk	Waffles w/ vanilla cream and cherry purée or fresh berries Tea or coffee w/ non-dairy milk	Mushroom/spinach tofu scramble w/ sliced avocados, WFPB toast w/ fruit purée Tea or coffee w/ non-dairy milk
Pumpkin nugget and tea	Puffed wheat w/ non-dairy milk	Avocado toast	Biscotti and tea
Veggie stir fry Fresh fruit	Dal w/ naan bread Salad	Veggie burger, potato salad, and watermelon mint salad	Pizza Fall kale salad
Crackers and/or veggies and hummus	Scones and cream Tea	Pumpkin pecan tart Tea	Baked potato w/ sour cream and green onions
Middle Eastern bowl w/ naan bread	Asian bowl Fresh fruit	Gyros w/ naan bread Salad	Chili w/ taco slaw and cornbread
Brazil nuts and apple sauce	Golden milk and biscotti	Fresh fruit and comfort tea	Sliced apple/ pumpkin bread

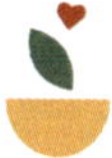

RESOURCES

The following resources were part, but not all of my research. I recommend getting audio recordings of the books. Because the research in some of them is extensive and might be easier to absorb while you are chopping veggies or making hummus. Each of the doctors has a different perspective and some of them have different chronic health conditions that they specialize in. For example, Dr. Esselstyn is a specialist in treating heart disease. Dr. Campbell spent much of his career researching and compiling research on diet and cancer. Each perspective is unique and valuable. You may want to follow most closely the recommendations of the doctor who is a specialist in any illnesses or conditions that you are most concerned with preventing or reversing.

BOOKS

The Starch Solution, John McDougall, M.D., Mary McDougall

The China Study, T. Colin Campbell, PhD., Thomas M. Campbell II, M.D.

How Not to Die, Michael Greger, M.D.

Prevent and Reverse Heart Disease: The Revolutionary, Scientifically Proven, Nutrition-Based Cure, Caldwell B. Esselstyn Jr. M.D.

Eat to Live, Joel Fuhrman, M.D.

Reversing Heart Disease, Dean Ornish, M.D.

VIDEOS

Forks over Knives

PlantPure Nation

Uprooting the Leading Causes of Death

WEBSITES

nutritionstudies.org

pcrm.org

nutritionfacts.org

forksoverknives.com

engine2diet.com

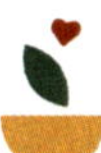

INDEX

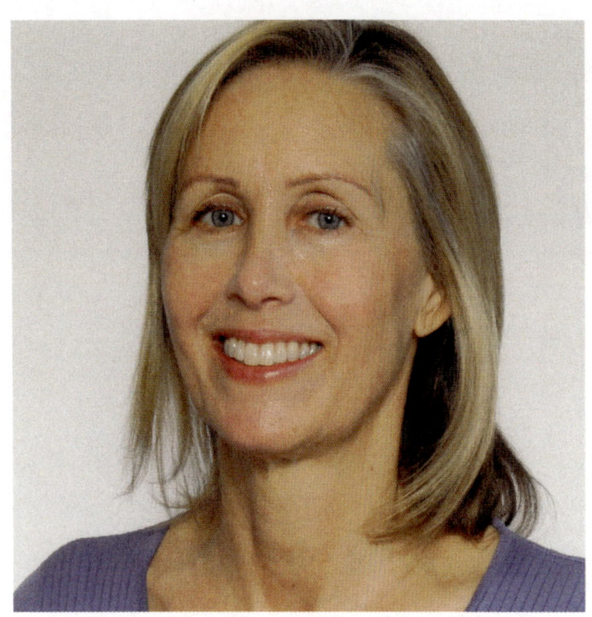

Elise Lovejoy is certified in Plant-based Nutrition by the Center for Nutrition Studies at eCornell and has a Master's degree in Education from Stanford. After a close family member was diagnosed with Stage IV cancer, she studied in depth the research of Doctors T. Colin Campbell, Caldwell B. Esselstyn Jr., Joel Furhman, Michael Greger, John McDougall, and Dean Ornish on the health benefits of a whole food, plant based diet. Having been on a whole food, plant based food plan for years, now, Elise is familiar with the challenges people face in making this diet and lifestyle change, and she is passionate about helping people successfully transition to WFPB eating and reap its benefits. Her goal with this book is to provide recipes that integrate the various perspectives of the doctors whose research she studied while offering a variety of comfort foods that will help the transition happen more naturally.

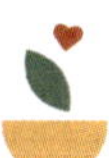

Made in the USA
San Bernardino, CA
26 May 2020